Psoriasis: A

Nicholas Lowe MD, FRCP
Clinical Professor of Dermatology,
UCLA School of Medicine,
California, USA
Senior Lecturer and Consultant in Dermatology,
University College London School of Medicine,
London, UK
and
The Cranley Clinic,
London, UK and
2001 Santa Monica Blvd,
California, USA

© Martin Dunitz Ltd 1998

First published in the United States in 1993 as *Managing your Psoriasis* by MasterMedia Ltd.

First published in the United Kingdom in 1998 by

Martin Dunitz Ltd
The Livery House
7– 9 Pratt Street
London NW1 0AE

A CIP record for this book is available from the British Library.

ISBN 1-85317-599-4

Printed and bound in Singapore by Kyodo Printing Co (S'pore) Pte Ltd.

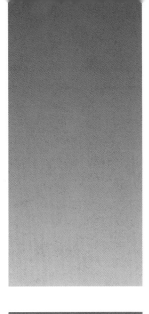

Contents

Acknowledgments

I want to give special thanks to my wife,
Pam, who has been a constant source of support in establishing and refining the
Southern California Dermatology and
Psoriasis Centres in California, USA and the
Cranley Clinic in London, England. She and
my daughters, Nichola and Philippa, have
given me the understanding and support that
have allowed me the time to complete this
project.

I want to especially acknowledge the many
lessons I have learned from my patients with
psoriasis. They have to live with a capricious,
unpredictable, emotionally draining and
occasionally disabling disease. They need our
understanding, support and encouragement.
It is important for them to know of progress
being made in the understanding and treatment of psoriasis so they may be encouraged
about new options for their treatment.

Foreword

This book meets the urgent need for a comprehensive, single-volume source of information on psoriasis for the public. Its complete review of the types of psoriasis and all the treatments provides the reader with an informative context by which to compare the merits of the various psoriasis treatment alternatives.

Improvements in technology and clinical research have improved the efficacy of traditional psoriasis therapies and generated new ones. We also have developed a greater understanding of what triggers psoriasis. Thousands of people with psoriasis have an improved quality of life as a result. Dr Lowe has been at the forefront of developing these new therapies and broadening our understanding of psoriasis. As a nationally recognized expert in treating this disorder, he has raised the standards in treating psoriasis. This book reflects his many years of experience in working with people to cope effectively with their psoriasis.

The National Psoriasis Foundation (USA) (NPF) was established by people living with psoriasis and their families as a volunteer, non-profit organization, to help people affected by psoriasis regain control of their lives. As knowledge is critical for anyone trying to cope successfully with psoriasis, the NPF places a high priority on education. Through its national membership newsletters and consumer booklets, NPF educates people about psoriasis and serves as a clearing- house for the latest information relating to treatment and research. Dr Lowe, as a member of the NPF's medical advisory board for many years, has been an important contributor to this national databank.

The Psoriasis Association in the UK and other psoriasis foundations and associations around the world provide self help information and education for people with psoriasis.

People living with psoriasis often find themselves on a frustrating quest for information about the disorder. This book responds to that need by providing a unique educational opportunity for the millions of Americans living with psoriasis to have easy access to information on psoriasis and the 'state of the art' in psoriasis therapy.

Gail M. Zimmerman
Executive Director,
National Psoriasis Foundation,
Portland, Oregon, USA

Introduction

Psoriasis has been recognized for centuries and it is likely that numerous disfiguring diseases, e.g. leprosy, have been confused with psoriasis. An early 1800s lithograph seen in *Figure 1* shows a medical artist's accurate picture of psoriasis at that time.

'The heartbreak of psoriasis'. For many millions of people around the world, this is more than an advertising slogan — it's a harsh reality of life. Psoriasis is one of the most common skin diseases, affecting one in 50 adults — and psoriasis is more than a physical malady. Its markings can make patients feel ashamed and unattractive, which can lead to psychological distress. And when the skin symptoms combine with related ailments like psoriatic arthritis, patients can understandably become depressed and disabled.

In the past, many psoriasis sufferers had to live with the knowledge that they could suffer an outbreak of their painful and uncomfortable disease at any time — usually the least convenient time. Many have become understandably frustrated with doctors they think cannot understand the

Figure 1
Lithograph of psoriasis.
An artist's impression of
a severe case.

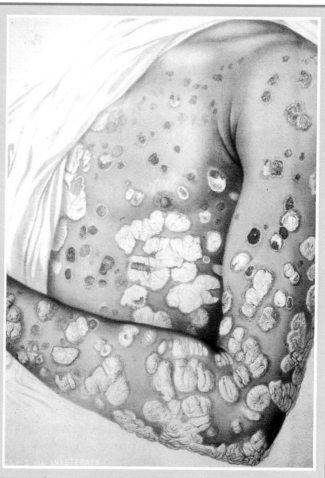

vagaries of their disease or don't care enough to find cures that really work safely.

But psoriasis treatments are changing. We in the medical community, and researchers in drug companies, are developing new treatments and improving old ones. Dermatologists have a clearer understanding than ever of how current treatments actually work. Until recently, we had proof that some of them worked, but no precise understanding of how. We also have a clearer understanding of how psoriasis develops. Once we understand its development fully, we will be able to stop the development process before the disease is full-blown — or even eliminate people's susceptibility to psoriasis altogether.

Several well-respected scientists are probing the possibility that genetic factors cause psoriasis. If researchers identify psoriasis-causing genes, they may be able to find ways to alter the gene so that it doesn't send psoriasis-causing messages to the skin. Once the stuff of horror movies and nightmares, genetic engineering is now the hook many researchers are hanging their most optimistic dreams on! Until a definitive cure is found,

knowledge of the increasingly good treatment options available can make a big difference in the daily life of a person with psoriasis.

This book is designed to provide understandable information about psoriasis, and I hope it will also serve to encourage patients who feel overwhelmed by their symptoms and their frustrations. In the following chapters, I will outline the different treatments currently available (both by prescription and over-the-counter) and discuss their benefits, drawbacks and proper uses. Newer treatments include novel vitamin A gels that can be combined with other therapies to provide increased improvement. There are effective ways to cope with psoriasis — successful ways to minimize the disease's discomforts and distresses. With appropriate medical treatment, psychological counselling, relaxation techniques, home therapy and the support of family and friends, you can reduce the impact of psoriasis, and lead a more comfortable, fulfilling life.

What is psoriasis?

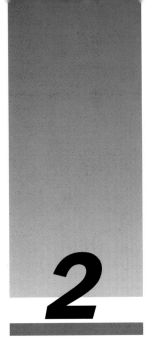

No one fully understands what causes psoriasis yet, but doctors have several theories. We have known for a long time that psoriasis seems to run in families. This is not to say that if you have the disease your children definitely will, or that if your parents didn't you won't either. Rather, there is a marked increase in psoriasis among people whose parents, grandparents or siblings have the disease. If one spouse has psoriasis, a couple's children have a one-in-four chance of developing psoriasis too. If both parents have psoriasis, there is a 50:50 chance that their children will inherit the disease. If one fraternal twin has psoriasis, there is a 70% chance that the other will, and there is a 90% chance that if one identical twin has the disease, so will the other.

Although we have nailed down the numbers, dermatologists and genetics experts still don't know exactly how psoriasis is passed from one generation to the next, but we are getting closer to an answer. Recent study of blood samples has suggested to researchers that there are several genes that transmit psoriasis. The exact locations of the genes remain unknown (there are millions of genes on each of the 26 chromosomes), but scientists are currently trying to identify them precisely, so that they can start experimenting with the genes and alter the way they affect people who are born with them.

Correct diagnosis of psoriasis

Proper diagnosis of your psoriasis helps to assure proper treatment. Many doctors who are not dermatologists see very few patients with psoriasis. Your family doctor may have difficulty in pin-pointing the diagnosis, which could lead to inappropriate treatment. That's why it is important to consult a dermatologist at the early stages of psoriasis.

The role of the dermatologist

Trained dermatologists can usually diagnose psoriasis simply by looking at the skin and other key areas like the nails and scalp, However, dermatologists may have a harder time diagnosing unusual instances of psoriasis or cases that have been incompletely treated by another doctor. Under these circumstances, the doctor may have to wait for you to develop more typical features of psoriasis before confirming the diagnosis.

In some cases, your dermatologist may suggest a skin biopsy to aid in the diagnosis. This is a very simple and relatively painless procedure. In a skin biopsy, the doctor takes very small samples of the skin, which has been numbed by a local anaesthetic. These samples can then be examined under the microscope and can reveal certain characteristics of psoriasis that will help the dermatologist to diagnose your psoriasis and devise a treatment plan that will work for you.

If your physician only treats mild cases of the disease, he or she may refer you to a psoriasis specialist or psoriasis centre where more advanced facilities are available.

Dermatologists can be supportive and positive when dealing with psoriasis. It is important for the psoriasis patient to realize that:

- *Many treatments are available to control their disease.*
- *Their disease can improve maximally or clear up for prolonged periods of time with the correct use of different treatments.*
- *The impact of the disease on their daily lives can be reduced significantly.*
- *Support groups, psychotherapy and counselling can lead to a major improvement in feelings of self-esteem and ability to cope with psoriasis.*
- *Improved treatments continue to be developed.*

The purpose of this book is to assist the psoriasis patient in dealing with their disease and to provide them with positive information about major improvements in the treatment of the disease which may result in many patients' lives being considerably improved over the next decade, as these new treatments become available.

There is no getting around the fact that psoriasis can be a difficult disease to live with. In moderate to severe cases, patients experience pain and severe discomfort. Their self-images can plummet. They understandably become tired of messy and sometimes smelly creams.

What causes psoriasis skin to look as it does?

Beyond understanding how psoriasis is inherited, researchers have several theories as to how psoriasis actually develops in people with a genetic predisposition to it. Recent research suggests several different possible sites (locations) for the 'psoriasis' gene — there may well be several genes. One theory is that a lack of control of the outer skin cells leads to the greatly increased production of cells that characterize psoriasis. This, in turn, may lead to an abnormality of the blood vessels and the inflammation characteristic of psoriasis.

Other researchers feel that psoriasis patients have an abnormality in the skin that leads to inflammation. This inflammation leads to a build-up of white blood cells from the blood. This build-up of white blood cells then triggers the thickened skin of psoriasis.

Still another possibility is that the epidermal skin cells fail to mature into the flat, thickened 'cornified' layer they're supposed to. As a result, the epidermis tries to produce more cells than usual, leading to the thickened epidermis, this then leads to inflammation.

A recent theory has suggested that there may be an abnormal immune reaction in skin with psoriasis. The precise abnormality is not known — it may be a lack of control of certain cells in the skin that regulate the immune system. This has been suggested because of the promising results doctors have obtained with the immune-regulating drug called Cyclosporine. Researchers believe that Cyclosporine may actually correct a local change of immunity in the skin. (I will discuss Cyclosporine in more detail in **Chapter 9**.)

Many patients find that symptoms vary over time. There are various reasons for this. First, infections may prompt or worsen psoriasis. For example, guttate psoriasis sometimes flares up in patients who are sensitive to bacterial (streptococcal) sore throats. Some people may get severe psoriasis on the skin-fold and scalp as a result of a yeast infection in the skin. Stress has also been named as a major culprit in psoriasis flare-ups. Fortunately, counselling and relaxation techniques can go a long way towards minimizing the stress trigger and can be very helpful in keeping psoriasis under control.

Let me stress that most people with psoriasis do NOT have immune deficiency, nor are they at increased risk of contracting AIDS. If there is an abnormal immune function in the skin, it is likely to affect only the skin. People with psoriasis do not display any evidence of general changes in their body's immunoregulatory systems.

Different types of psoriasis

Psoriasis reveals itself in many ways. The following are the most common varieties.

Common plaque (patch) psoriasis

Common psoriasis, also known as psoriasis vulgaris, is by far the most common type of psoriasis, accounting for 80–90% of all psoriasis patients. It appears as raised red scaling patches. The scales, which are often silvery and thickened, appear most frequently on the

elbows, knees, scalp and lower back. *Figure 2* shows a typical elbow patch. However, all parts of the skin may occasionally be subject to psoriasis.

Guttate psoriasis

This type of psoriasis often starts in childhood or teenage years, with the sudden onset of small, raindrop-like patches of scaling skin ('guttate'), much thinner than plaque psoriasis. Often a sore throat caused by streptococcal infection will prompt the appearance of guttate psoriasis. (See the case study of Lillian in *Chapter 11* as an example.)

Guttate psoriasis *(see Figure 3)* often covers large parts of the body, but it responds rapidly to ultraviolet therapy and some other forms of treatment. It can also clear up, leaving the patient free of further outbreaks of guttate psoriasis. In such cases, localized patches or plaques of psoriasis may develop later in life.

Skin-fold, 'flexural' and genital psoriasis

This type of psoriasis occurs in the skin-folds or flexures and can cause great discomfort when one part of the skin rubs against another. This discomfort can be so severe as to become disabling for the patient. It can occur in genital areas, which can lead to

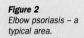

Figure 2
Elbow psoriasis – a typical area.

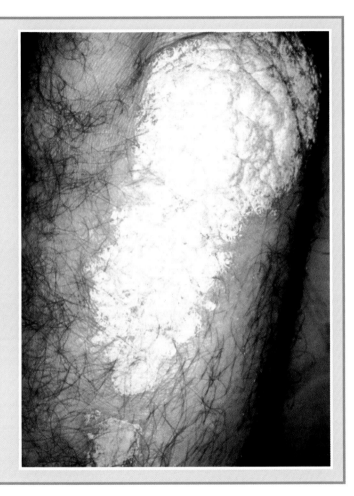

Figure 3
A patient treated with oral acitretin and ultraviolet (UVB) treatment. Before (a) and after (b) 8 weeks. He then started to reduce his dose of acitretin gradually over 4 weeks. Ultraviolet was continued once-a-week as a 'maintenance' treatment.

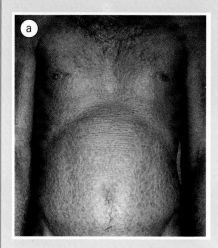
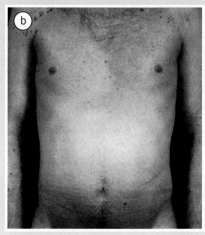

discomfort and difficulties with sexual relations. It is more common and troublesome in overweight patients.

Erythrodermic or exfoliative psoriasis

When psoriasis completely covers the body, it is known as erythrodermic, exfoliative psoriasis or generalized psoriasis. Because such a large area of skin is involved, patients may feel extreme discomfort. Patients may also encounter problems controlling their body temperature, particularly in very hot or very cold climates. Older people, particularly those with heart disease and heart failure, can also develop problems from accelerated heart rate due to increased blood supply flowing through the severely inflamed skin. This may lead to heart failure.

Pustular psoriasis

Localized pustular psoriasis

An unusual form of the disease, pustular psoriasis is often found on the palms of the hands or the soles of the feet. It can be very uncomfortable when you are working with your hands or walking. Instead of thickened scaling patches, patients often see brownish or whitish dots surrounded by inflamed red skin. Some patients with pustular psoriasis also have plaques and patches of regular psoriasis.

Standard psoriasis treatments must be modified to treat pustular psoriasis. For example, topical cortisones on the hands and feet usually have to be covered with plastic gloves or plastic wrap to enable sufficient medication to penetrate the thickened skin of the palms and soles.

Generalized pustular psoriasis

This is a very severe form of psoriasis in which the skin is covered with non-infected pustules, which are collections of white blood cells appearing in the skin. Patients feel very ill and frequently have fever. General pustular psoriasis of this type may be caused by a number of things, including infections, medications like lithium, or the use of systemic cortisones. It may also occur as a reaction to severe sunburn. *Figure 4* shows generalised pustular psoriasis and its response to treatment.

Generalized pustular psoriasis requires urgent dermatological care. Fortunately, though, this form of the disease is rare.

DIFFERENT TYPES OF PSORIASIS

Common, plaque type

Guttate

Flexural

Erythrodermic (rare)

Pustular (rare)

Figure 4
Severe or generalized pustular psoriasis. Before (a) and after (b) 10 days of systemic retinoid treatment. The optimum treatment now for this type of psoriasis is oral acitretin.

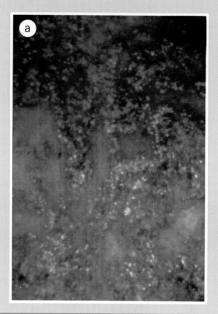
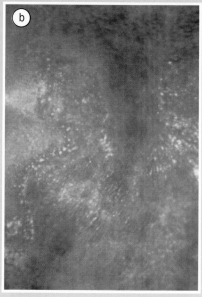

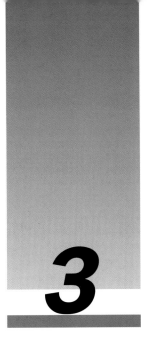

Learning to live with psoriasis — coping mechanisms and programmes

3

Our understanding of psoriasis is increasing but as yet we have no cure for this once baffling disease. However, until a cure is found, there are many treatments, strategies and attitudes that can make life easier and less painful for psoriasis patients.

If you have suffered from psoriasis for a while, you probably know that stress can aggravate the condition. Avoiding stress is difficult for anyone living at the end of the twentieth century, but to make matters worse, psoriasis itself can heighten stress, creating a vicious cycle of flare-ups and increased tension. Also, once the cycle has built up momentum, it can affect your self-esteem and can even cause problems at work and in your social life.

Luckily, there are several ways to avoid or minimize the stresses that life and psoriasis bring with them, and more stress-minimizers are being developed every day.

Stress reduction and psoriasis

There are several ways to ease the stresses psoriasis brings with it:

- *Make your friends and colleagues aware of your condition, and let them know how they can help you through the tough times. If you don't ask for support, no one will know that you need it. Enlisting friends' support is helpful not only on a practical level, but also because it will make you feel less alone in your disease.*

- *If you find that your psoriasis worsens at certain times of the year, avoid making big time commitments for those periods. Try to reduce the number of deadlines you face and don't plan large gatherings or social events at home. It is essential that you have sufficient time to unwind and relax during psoriasis outbreaks.*

- *Don't rely on drugs or alcohol to lift you out of the depression that sometimes accompanies psoriasis. For one thing, while these substances might improve your mood temporarily, they may lead to even greater depression the morning after. Also, alcohol can be dangerous when taken in combination with some of the drugs used to treat severe psoriasis.*

- *Start the day with pleasant thoughts and images. Imagine that your skin is going to improve and think about the positive aspects of your life. Picture yourself in a peaceful and tranquil setting, or listen to a tape of crashing waves or rain-forest noises. Relaxation tapes are available at many music stores.*

If you find that your psoriasis is stressing you out even with all of these exercises or that everyday stresses are making it worse, your first step should be to visit your dermatologist. Dermatologists can be supportive and helpful when dealing with psoriasis, and dermatologists have a lot to be positive about today. Many new treatments are available to control psoriasis and with correct use of these treatments, your psoriasis can improve maximally or clear for prolonged periods of time. Learning about these treatments may help you not only tackle the physical symptoms of your condition, but may also give you an emotional boost. Just knowing that help is on the way can be very helpful in itself!

Discussing your psoriasis and its effects with a dermatologist who understands them can go a long way to relieving anxiety, but more importantly, your dermatologist can recommend the stress-relief techniques that will work best in getting your psoriasis under control. He or she may refer you to a psychotherapist for talk therapy, stress reduction programmes and biofeedback. In addition to reducing the stress that can aggravate psoriasis, psychotherapy may help you to change your responses to the psoriasis itself. Working with a good psychotherapist, you will be able to learn new behaviour patterns that can enable you to cope more effectively with your emotional concerns and to control the effect psoriasis has on your social interactions, rather than letting the disease control you.

Consider joining a support group

If you would like to discuss the stresses that lead to and come from psoriasis outbreaks, you may want to join a support group, instead of or in addition to one-to-one psychotherapy. In a room full of other psoriasis patients, you will soon discover that you are not the only person who is afraid or embarrassed to go to the beach. You will learn that there are others who feel awkward about exposing their skin, even to close friends and family. Most importantly, you'll learn that there are ways to overcome or minimize these negative feelings and pump up your self-esteem. The best support groups are usually led by a patient, doctor or psychologist who

can guide all the members toward a more optimistic outlook, and support groups are most supportive when they meet frequently and are limited to about 10 people. Listening to a few people speak in a huge group might be marginally helpful, but group meetings are most effective when they are small enough for you to voice your feelings and concerns every time you meet and get individual feedback from the other members.

Psychotherapy support

As you discuss the stresses in your life with your psychotherapist or your support group members, you may learn first-hand what dermatologists have known for a while — often several weeks elapse between the time of the stress and the worsening of the psoriasis. You may have thought that there was no connection between life's little dramas and the state of your skin. But, when you come to see the cycle's pattern, it will be easier for you to break the cycle. For example, if you discover that having a fight with your parent, child, spouse or work supervisor always results in a bad psoriatic outbreak, you may have an extra incentive to find a more amicable way to settle your differences. If nothing else, recognizing exactly how and when stress affects your psoriasis will help you to find the relaxation techniques that help minimize the flare-ups if you employ them soon enough after the stress trigger.

Some of the techniques that may work for you include self-hypnosis, meditation and yoga. Major metropolitan centres have classes in all of these disciplines, and some psoriasis centres have support groups that can train you in these stress reduction techniques as well.

If these stress reduction strategies are not sufficient, you may want to consult a psychiatrist. Unlike psychologists, psychiatrists are licensed to prescribe drugs, and there are many new forms of drug therapy that are designed to reduce stress and depression. However, let me stress that these drugs must be used under the continued guidance of a psychiatrist, because there are sometimes side-effects to be weighed against the benefits of the drug. Some of the medicines now available include Prozac and its relatives, which are anti-anxiety, anti-panic and anti-depressant drugs, and Buspar, also an antidepressant. Your doctor or psychiatrist can tell you more about specific drugs and their respective pros and cons.

In the years I have been treating psoriasis, I have found that the patients who have been most successful in dealing with psoriasis, and

by successful I mean in their attitudes as well as in their physical conditions, share several characteristics. First, they have made peace with their psoriasis. This doesn't mean that they have given up on seeking treatments that work for them. On the contrary, it means that they have said to themselves, 'I have psoriasis. I will not be ashamed of it or limited by it, either socially or professionally. Since I cannot change it, I will accept it and continue to treat it as best I can'.

This leads us to the second main characteristic: the most successful patients are persistent in their treatments. It can become quite discouraging for patients to live through so many new psoriatic eruptions, especially after relishing the freedom of being clear for a few weeks or months. Unfortunately, this is often the nature of psoriasis. The patients who cope best are those who know to expect that new outbreaks may occur and are willing to try new treatments, creams, shampoos and whatever else may be required.

As you continue to read this book and to live with psoriasis, remember that you may not be able to control your skin, but you can control your attitude towards it. Accepting psoriasis as a fact of life will free up your emotional energy for more productive endeavours and should alleviate some of the stress associated with psoriasis.

Psoriasis in special sites: scalp, nail, skin-fold and genitals — special treatments and care required

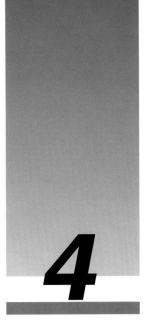

Scalp psoriasis

Scalp psoriasis, which occurs when excessive scaling occurs together with inflammation, affects at least half of all psoriasis patients *(Figure 5)*. Because scales on the scalp, face and clothing can be very obvious, this ailment can be very rough on a patient's emotional and psychological well-being. Some patients even try to scrape their severe scaling off. Don't be one of them! Scraping damages the scalp skin and worsens psoriasis.

There is good news and bad news regarding scalp psoriasis. The good news is that with so many treatment options available, most patients can be helped. The bad news is that the scalp is one of the most difficult areas to treat, and many patients do not easily tolerate the treatment agents. Thus, frequent alterations in their medication plans are needed. It is a constant challenge to clear scalp psoriasis effectively, maintain improvements and modify treatments based on patients' reactions to the toxicity of medications.

Figure 5
Scalp psoriasis. Showing psoriasis (a). Before (b) and after (c) Cortisone lotion plus coal tar shampoos daily.
Scalp products (d) and shampoos (e) and (f).

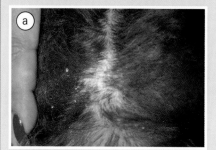
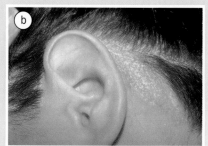
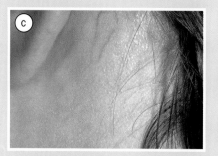
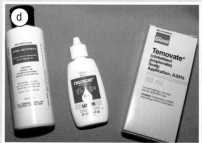
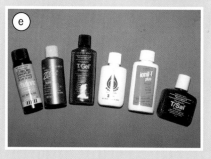
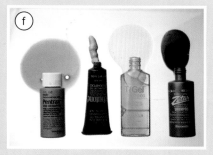

There are a few conditions that mimic the symptoms of scalp psoriasis, but they are actually different diseases. Seborrhoeic dermatitis or seborrhoeic eczema of the scalp is probably the most common condition that looks like scalp psoriasis. If your dermatologist has prescribed Anthralin be sure that someone in the clinic (usually it's a nurse) gives you detailed how-to's, so that you can avoid unnecessary staining and irritation. Most importantly, remember to shampoo backwards, away from the face, to prevent the Anthralin from dripping onto your forehead and from there into your eyes.

Imidazole lotions or creams are effective for some patients and once they have achieved maximum improvement, patients can usually reduce their applications from daily to occasional use and still effectively control their psoriasis.

Cortisone-containing scalp preparations are frequently helpful *(Figure 5d)*. Injecting cortisone directly into the lesions of scalp psoriasis can lead to long periods of improvement for some patients with tough but localized cases. PUVA (Psoralen-ultraviolet-A) therapy may help — particularly with thin-haired patients — and sunlight therapy is sometimes effective as well.

I believe that shampoos are vitally important in controlling scalp psoriasis, even though there have been few scientific studies on them. Therapeutic shampoos, usually available without a doctor's prescription, usually contain coal tars, wood tars, salicylic acid, sulphur, selenium and zinc parathione or they may combine several of these agents in one shampoo. I give samples of several shampoos to my patients and allow them to select one that proves most beneficial and least irritating. I have found that some patients with blonde or dyed hair resist using tar shampoos because they sometimes stain the hair. As these shampoos can be expensive, one of my patients offered the following tip to reduce the cost.

'I apply tar soap (Polytar) as the first coat. I then apply the tar shampoo such as T-Sal, T-gel or Pentrax which are highly concentrated and require smaller quantities. A bar of tar soap lasts a very long time. For me, regular cream rinse works very well, and I prefer it to the costly dermatological products.'

Newer, less messy scalp treatments

A prescription shampoo called Nizoral contains ketoconazole to reduce yeasts present on scalp skin, which in turn may improve scalp psoriasis in some patients.

Tazarotene gel (known as Tazorac in the USA and Canada and Zorac in Europe) applied to the scalp nightly or on alternate nights is very helpful in improving psoriasis. Some patients also benefit from Dovonex scalp solution.

Scalp treatments

> **SOME PREPARATIONS FOR TREATING SCALP PSORIASIS THAT ARE AVAILABLE IN USA:**
>
> **Steroid preparations**
> Aristocort Lotion
> Cordran Lotion
> Cyclicort Lotion
> Dermasmoothe FS Lotion
> Diprolene Gel
> Diprolene Lotion
> Diprosone Lotion
> Lidex Gel
> Temovate Lotion
> Valisone Lotion
>
> **Purified tar preparations**
> Aquator Gel
> Baker's P and S Plus Gel
> Estar Tar Gel
> Fototar Tar Cream
> Psorigel
> T-Derm Tar and Salicylic Acid Scalp
>   Lotion
> T-Derm Tar Oil
>
> **Salicylic acid preparations**
> Keralyt Gel

> **Other preparations**
> P and S Liquid
> Dovonex Scalp Lotion
> Tazorac Gel
>
> **AND IN EUROPE:**
>
> Betacap Scalp
> Bettamouse Scalp
> Betnovate Lotion
> Dermavate Scalp
> Diprosone Lotion
> Diposalic Scalp
> Dovonex Scalp Lotion
> Elocon Lotion
> Locoid Scalp
> Stredlex Lotion
> Zorac Gel

A shower cap can be used to cover the scalp after applying the treatments at night *(Figure 6).*

The treatments outlined in the Box are recommended for localized scalp psoriasis as well as for the more generalized disease. In serious cases, you may want to go to a treatment centre equipped to apply thick preparations and to remove them with specialized detergents. Our treatment centre in Southern California offers scalp therapy, combining topical lotions and therapeutic shampoos.

Patients with severe and stubborn scalp psoriasis have benefited greatly from a systemic therapy that utilizes methotrexate,

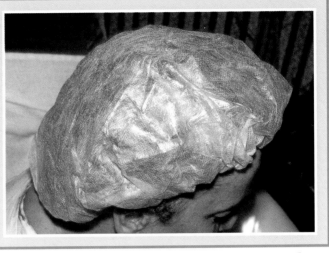

Figure 6
A scalp cap will help the lotion to work and protect your pillows.

retinoids or Cyclosporine (see *Chapter 9* for more on these).

In all but the most severe cases, scalp psoriasis can be improved. It may take patience and persistence to find the right formula, but the results are well worth waiting for.

Nail psoriasis

Nail psoriasis affects almost half of all people with psoriasis and 80% of those with psoriatic arthritis. Patients complain about changes in the appearance and texture of the fingernails more often than toenails, but this may be because patients are less likely to notice or be bothered by toenail psoriasis. Some people have psoriasis on their nails but nowhere else. *Figures 7a and b and Figure 8* show different degrees of nail psoriasis.

In severe cases of nail psoriasis a person can actually become disabled when trying to use their hands or fingers, and even mild cases can cause some disfigurement. Psoriatic nails may lose their normal, healthy look and can become yellowed or otherwise discoloured. The most frequent symptom of nail psoriasis is the appearance of pits. These are shallow depressions that are usually less than 1mm in diameter. There may be a few isolated pits on one or two nails or on all nails.

Figure 7
(a) Mild nail psoriasis. Notice the little 'dells' or 'pits'. (b) More severe nail psoriasis. The nails are roughened, irregular and discoloured.

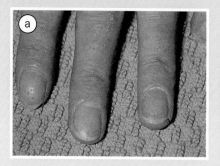
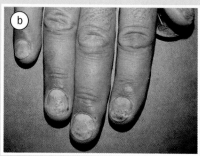

Figure 8
Moderately severe nail psoriasis showing noticeable nail psoriasis, lifting of nails and pitting.

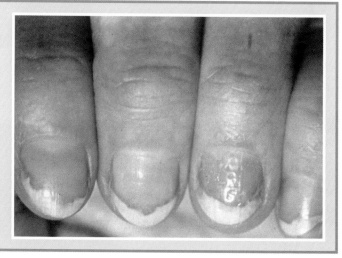

Extensive nail psoriasis can actually cause the nails to crumble easily. Other symptoms include furrows, roughness and grooving. Nails sometimes detach themselves from the nail-bed. This condition is called onycholysis. This occurs almost as often as pitting. Usually, the nail detachment begins at the edge of the nail and may spread backwards under it. The area surrounding the onycholysis may have yellowed or become brownish and can have the appearance of oil spots.

If a bacterial or fungal infection emerges in psoriatic nails, you may experience more painful swelling of the skin around the nail.

Unfortunately, nearly every method of local nail treatment has disadvantages. Injectable cortisones sometimes work, but the injections can be uncomfortable and there are also the possibilities of relapses and skin atrophy (thinned skin). Patients opting for injections usually need at least one injection every month for 3–4 months.

High-potency topical steroids applied under the nail may also help, but this kind of therapy must be continued for several months because nails grow slowly. Furthermore, soft tissue under the nail can atrophy before any normal nail growth emerges.

Tazorac gel applied around and under the nails at night, alternated with a good

moisturizing cream, may be helpful for nail psoriasis.

Sometimes, nail psoriasis can go away all by itself. My general advice for psoriasis patients with nail disease is to try to avoid damage and injury to the nails which could prompt or worsen nail psoriasis problems.

IF YOU HAVE NAIL PSORIASIS, TRY TO FOLLOW THESE RECOMMENDATIONS:

- *Keep nails trimmed down to where the nail is firmly attached. This avoids putting pressure on loose nails.*
- *Avoid activities that might injure the nails.*
- *Wear gloves when working with your hands.*
- *Try to improve the appearance of damaged nails with artificial nails, clear or coloured nail varnish.*
- *See your dermatologist for advice if the nails or surrounding skin becomes too uncomfortable.*

Skin-fold and genital psoriasis

When psoriasis affects skin sites such as underarms, groin and genital skin, patients may become extremely uncomfortable and often suffer considerable pain and embarrassment in intimate situations. Fortunately, several treatment options are available. These skin areas are very prone to irritation from some topical medications and dermatologists must use extreme caution when prescribing treatments.

My recommendations for treating these delicate skin areas include using only mild cortisone creams or ointments, with none stronger than 1% hydrocortisone. These may be combined with antifungal and anti-yeast creams, because these skin areas can easily become infected with yeast such as Candida and fungi.

I avoid suggesting coal tar preparations because of the possible risk of skin cancer if they are used long term in skin-fold areas, particularly on genital skin. Instead, I suggest that patients shampoo these sites when showering. Use a shampoo containing salicylic acid or sulphur, for example, Sebulex or Nizoral.

Creams that reduce skin yeasts may also improve psoriasis — examples are Nizoral cream (USA and Europe) and Daktacort cream (UK).

For more severe cases, I recommend therapy at a treatment centre with higher strength steroid anti-yeast creams, such as Lotrisone. These can be used for short time periods, but should be avoided long term because the strong steroid may cause skin thinning.

Use of Dovonex cream or Tazorac gel (usually 0.05%) is sometimes valuable. If they irritate the skin-fold or genital skin, reduce application frequency or stop them.

When psoriasis affects the genital skin, both the patient and his or her sexual partner may need reassurance and encouragement. If you and your spouse or partner are concerned or put off by genital psoriasis, talk to your dermatologist together.

Remember: psoriasis is not infectious and cannot be transmitted to another person by sexual contact. Using condoms may be helpful for male patients with psoriasis on their penis and women can use lubricating jelly to reduce aggravating their genital psoriasis during sexual intercourse.

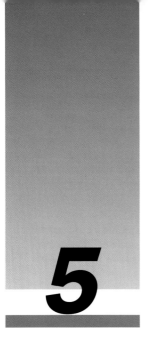

Psoriatic arthritis

Psoriatic arthritis, which affects about 10% of all psoriasis patients, most commonly flares up in the hands and feet. It can also cause inflammation, swelling and pain in larger joints, including the knees, elbows and hips, and the spine. Like all arthritis, psoriatic arthritis causes stiffness, pain and lack of movement in affected areas.

Psoriatic arthritis can occur in adults or children. In the vast majority (84%) of adults who have the condition, psoriasis alone precedes the onset of arthritis, sometimes by as much as 20 years. The skin and joints become afflicted simultaneously about 10% of the time and often nails are affected as well.

In children, arthritis precedes psoriasis in up to 52% of all cases, with girls contracting psoriatic arthritis nearly three times as often as boys.

We do not know why some patients with psoriasis get arthritis. Patients who develop psoriatic arthritis in their backs, a condition known as spondylitis, often have an inherited risk for back arthritis. Other types of psoriatic arthritis do not have this hereditary link. Scientists are trying to understand the link between arthritis and psoriasis more clearly. One study shows that people with severe skin psoriasis have a greater propensity towards arthritis and another study indicates that patients with pustular psoriasis were likely to develop more severe psoriatic arthritis. In fact, many psoriatics find that their arthritis is more severe than their skin disease.

There are several main types of psoriatic arthritis afflicting adults.

Treatment of psoriatic arthritis

It is ideal for patients with psoriatic arthritis and psoriasis to be under a rheumatologist's care for their arthritis, and see a dermatologist separately for their skin disease. Improving and controlling the skin disease often helps the arthritis as well.

As extensive skin psoriasis can be emotionally debilitating in itself, the additional burden of arthritis can become devastating. Therefore, managing the skin, the joints and the psyche are critical in an overall treatment plan. A number of treatment options are now available.

Patients suffering from prolonged joint stiffness, pain, fatigue and joint swelling need rest. Sometimes activity splints are helpful, these enable patients to maintain some function in their hands. Alternatively, rest splints protect the joints and help ease inflammation and other symptoms.

Nonsteroidal anti-inflammatory drugs (NSAIDS) provide relief by reducing inflammation and pain in the joints. There are several NSAIDs available, including aspirin, but none will prompt a remission of the disease, and some may have side-effects.

NONSTEROIDAL ANTI-INFLAMMATORY (ARTHRITIS) DRUGS:

USA
Meclomen
Clinoral
Motrin
Naprosyn, Anaprox
Tolectin
Voltaren

Less commonly used
Feldene
Azulfidine

EUROPE
Brufen
Clinoril
Feldene
Indomid
Motrin
Orudis
Voltarol

'Remittive' agents

If the psoriatic arthritis has become severe, your doctor may prescribe drugs to try and protect the joints from further destruction.

Methotrexate, which will be discussed later, is frequently used to treat other cases of severe psoriasis as well as to manage psoriatic arthritis. (See **Chapter 9** for more details about methotrexate.) Other treatments for psoriatic arthritis are listed as follows.

Cyclosporine by mouth may also be prescribed for severe psoriasis and arthritis *(see Figure 9)*.

Gold

Yes, gold. This precious metal can be injected into a muscle or taken orally and may be very valuable for some patients with psoriatic arthritis. Skin rashes may flare up as a side-effect, though. Your doctor will have to monitor your blood pressure and kidney function.

> *SOME SIDE-EFFECTS OF NONSTEROIDAL ANTI-INFLAMMATORY DRUGS INCLUDE:*
> * *Kidney problems*
> * *Skin rashes*
> * *Sun sensitivity*

> * *Stomach pains and heartburn*
> * *Bleeding from the upper bowel*
> * *Worsening of psoriasis (occasionally with indomethacin)*

Antimalarial drugs

Antimalarial drugs, such as chloroquine, hydroxychloroquine and atabrine, can be very useful for patients with psoriatic arthritis.

Systemic corticosteroids

Systemic corticosteroids are usually not recommended in the management of psoriatic arthritis because while they may ease symptoms, these drugs do not stop the disease's progression. When systemic corticosteroids are stopped, the skin psoriasis may get severely worse, occasionally turning into generalized pustular or exfoliative psoriasis.

Injections and orthopaedic surgery

Local steroids, however, can be very effective when injected into inflamed joints or tendons. Joint surgery may be helpful to some patients who have deforming types of arthritis, for example, on the fingers and toes, but only when the active, inflamed stages of the arthritis subside.

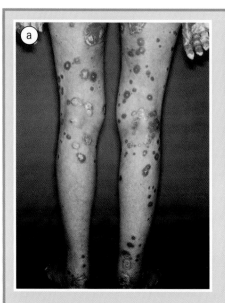
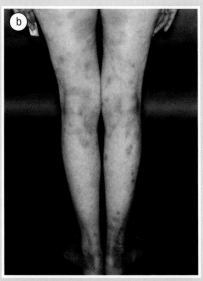
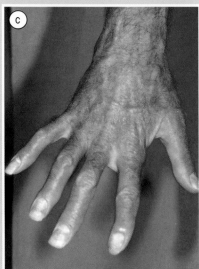

Figure 9
A patient with severe psoriasis and arthritis of her
hands. Before (a) and after (b) 6 weeks of treatment
with Cyclosporine by mouth. The Cyclosporine dose was
gradually reduced and the patient was then treated
with low dosage methotrexate once-a-week by mouth
and ultraviolet therapy. (c) Psoriatic arthritis of hands.

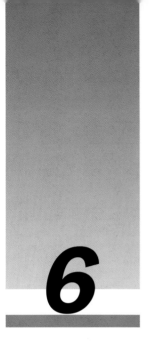

Children with psoriasis

Psoriasis may appear as early as birth. In fact, 10–15% of all psoriasis patients first encountered their skin condition before the age of 10, and 30% before the age of 20. More girls get psoriasis than boys, although the male/female ratio is about equal in adults.

Parents who have psoriasis themselves sometimes feel guilty when their children develop it and many psoriatics agonize over whether to have children at all, fearing that their offspring will experience the same discomfort, pain and embarrassment they have endured. But while childhood psoriasis can be uncomfortable and embarrassing, it is also usually treatable. Identifying and understanding your child's disease are the first steps to helping him or her live with it and flourish despite the discomforts and inconveniences of psoriasis.

Common forms of childhood psoriasis

Along with the usual appearance of plaques, children also develop guttate psoriasis *(see Figure 10)*, often preceded by an upper respiratory infection or streptococcal infection —

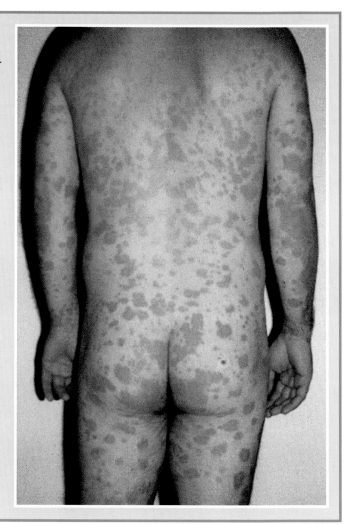

Figure 10
'Guttate' psoriasis –
a type often seen in
children and teenagers.
It may occur following
a sore throat.

also known as strep throat. Seek a paediatrician's care for these infections while you continue to take your child to the dermatologist for treatment of any skin symptoms.

Children are also particularly prone to seborrhoeic psoriasis and scalp psoriasis. Some infants are troubled by psoriasis in the usual 'diaper rash' zones.

Dermatologists should use caution in prescribing a treatment plan for children, as the disease may persist throughout a lifetime and will vary in severity. High-potency topical steroids should be avoided. A medium-strength steroid is the highest dosage I would recommend for children. 'Old' treatments such as coal tar ointments and Anthralin (Dithranol) can be used with supervision in children. 'New' treatments like Dovonex and Tazorac gel can also be safely employed.

I believe strongly that children with more severe psoriasis who fail to respond to these recommended topical treatments should be treated at a day-care centre when such facilities are available.

Fortunately, very few children develop severe and life-threatening psoriatic conditions. In the rare instances where it does occur, great care must be taken in selecting treatment. A short course of systemic retinoids is justified only for severe, uncontrolled erythroderma or generalized pustular psoriasis. In any case, systemic retinoid therapy should not be prolonged in children. PUVA therapy may be useful in treating severe psoriasis in children, but again, only for short periods because of the risk of skin cancer. Parents (or prospective parents) who worry about their children becoming psoriatics should remind themselves that psoriasis sometimes disappears on its own and those that do have it can have long, successful remissions. Furthermore, the condition can be managed very well with proper therapy.

In the meantime, there are things that parents can do to help support their children through their psoriatic episodes.

HELPING CHILDREN WITH PSORIASIS

- *Telephone your child's teacher or make an appointment to discuss the child's condition. Make sure that the teacher understands that psoriasis is not contagious. Find out how other children are treating your child and ask the teacher to speak to any children who may fear or not understand why your child looks different. If other kids are picking on your child, you may want to call their parents personally.*

- Set a positive example for your child. When others ask questions about psoriasis, discuss it matter-of-factly without any shame or embarrassment. If you accept the condition as an objective fact, so will your child.

- For younger children, add some 'play time' into medication time. Play games with ointments, (connect the dots to draw pictures, for example). Sing songs, talk about pleasant experiences the child has or is looking forward to and give your full attention to the child. Listen to his objections when he voices them and remain sympathetic but firm about applying the prescribed medications. Try to relax with your child during these application sessions.

- Explain to your child that everyone has problems or imperfections — some are visible and others are not. Help an older child find a hero who has overcome a physical challenge and read a book about that person.

- The Psoriasis Association in the UK (01604 711129) has a series of helpful pamphlets for psoriasis patients and their families.

- The National Psoriasis Foundation in the USA (NPF) has a 10-minute video called Kids With Psoriasis Need Friends Too. To purchase the tape or rent it write to NPF, 6600 SW, 92nd Avenue, Suite 300, Portland, OR 97223, USA. You can also arrange to show the tape to your child's class, particularly if peer questions and teasing have been bothering your child.

- The NPF also has a pen-pal network for children who would enjoy correspondence with another child with psoriasis. Write to the above address for more information.

- Try to live life as normally as possible and minimize the impact the child's psoriasis has on the family. Don't worry excessively about future episodes or how severe they will be. Take one day at a time.

Topical therapy: steroids, tars, dithranol, vitamin A- and D-related creams, lotions and gels

Somethings old, somethings new

There are dozens of topical agents available to help treat psoriasis. These include steroids, tars, keratolytics and Anthralin (Dithranol) moisturizers. Recent new treatments are the vitamin D topicals (Dovonex cream, ointment and lotion) and vitamin A gels (Tazorac/Zorac). This chapter will tell you a little about each of these and will help you understand when the use of a particular topical agent is called for.

Topical steroids: corticosteroids and cortisones

Steroids can be applied as ointments, creams, lotions, aerosols or tapes. Your dermatologist will decide on the type, potency and frequency of a steroid based on your particular condition.

Thick, plaque-type psoriasis on elbows, knees, palms, soles and other thickly skinned areas tend to resist steroids and require other topical therapy. Alternatively, lesions in body folds, the groin area, eyelids and other thinly skinned areas are usually more sensitive to steroid treatment. Topical steroids can be used to complement other forms of topical therapy, such as tar and ultraviolet light or Tazorac gel, but they are not meant to replace them. Your dermatologist will select a steroid based on the location and severity of the lesion and the steroid's strength. *Figure 11* shows the results of combining a strong cortisone cream plus an alpha hydroxy acid lotion.

Be careful when using topical steroids, they are expensive and quite potent and must be applied only as directed by a doctor. Some patients misuse steroids, rubbing too much of the medication into their skin. They think that if a little is good, a lot must be better. This is absolutely not true! Use your medication sparingly and apply only to the areas directed.

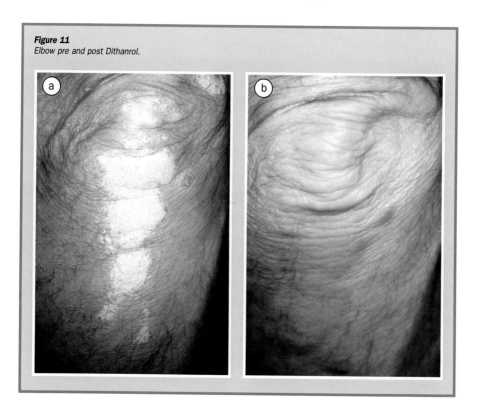

Figure 11
Elbow pre and post Dithanrol.

Strong steroids should not be applied to the face or skin-folds unless otherwise directed. Should any new skin irritation, bruising, ulcers or skin infections occur, *stop the treatment until you have consulted your doctor.*

Given their potency, it comes as no surprise that topical steroids have side-effects, which increase with the use of extremely strong agents. Fortunately, most of these side-effects can be handled either by discontinuing the steroid or by introducing another medication.

Side-effects are also more likely where the skin being treated is inherently thin, but even thicker skin may atrophy (become very thin),

(See Figure 12). This condition can sometimes be reversed once the medication has been stopped. Thinning skin is a particular problem with babies and young children, because their skin is naturally thin. As a result, most dermatologists will try to avoid long-term application of strong topical steroids in young patients.

Other side-effects of steroids include acne, rosacea, secondary infections of the skin and dermatitis. Glaucoma (increased eye pressure) may result from the use of topical steroids close to the eye. Only the weakest steroid agents should be used near the eye and then, only for limited amounts of time.

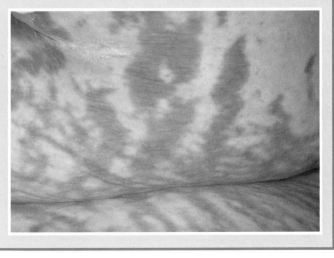

Figure 12
Skin thinning from the use of strong cortisone-containing cream over several years. These creams are very useful for short (several weeks) periods to avoid skin thinning.

**TIPS FOR USING TOPICAL STEROIDS —
CREAM, GELS, LOTIONS, TAPES**

- Apply the steroid to the skin lesion in
a thin film, with your fingertip — use
sparingly

- Never use someone else's steroids

- Steroids range from mild to very
potent — always know the potency of
your medication

- Use the steroids only on skin areas
your doctor prescribed them for. Do
not, for example, apply a steroid
intended for the knees to the face or
groin area

- Avoid applying stronger steroids to
face and skin-folds

Ratings of topical steroid strength (USA and UK)

Table 1
Topical corticosteroids currently available

Group I strongest – Group VII weakest USA	UK
Group I	**Group I**
Diprolene ointment 0.5%	Demovate
Diprolene gel	Demovate NN
Psorcon ointment	Halciderm
Temovate cream	Nerisonetate
Temovate ointment	**Group II**
Temovate lotion	Adcortyl
Ultravate cream	Aureocoor
Ultravate ointment	Betnovate
Group II	Cultivate
Cyclocort ointment 0.1%	Diprosalve
Diprosone ointment 0.05%	Elocon
Florone ointment 0.05%	Fucibet
Halog ointment 0.05%	Locoid
Lidex cream 0.1%	Nerisone
Lidex ointment 0.05%	Propaderm
Maxivate cream	Synalar
Maxivate ointment	Tricloityl
Maxiflor ointment 0.05%	
Topicort cream 0.25%	
Topicort ointment 0.25%	
Topsyn gel 0.05%	

USA	UK
Group III	**Group III**
Aristocort cream (III) 0.5%	Alphaderm
Diprosome cream 0.05%	Calmcoid HC
Florone cream 0.05%	Eumovate
Maxiflor cream 0.05%	Haelan
Valisone ointment 0.1%	Modvasone
Group IV	Synalar 1:4
Aristocort cream 0.1%	Trimovate
Benisone ointment 0.025%	Ultralanum
Cordran ointment 0.05%	**Group IV**
Kenalog ointment 0.1%	Alphosyl HC
Synalar cream (HP) 0.2%	Carbocort
Synalar ointment 0.025%	Cobadex
Topicort LP cream 0.05%	Daktacort
Group V	Dioderm
Benisone cream 0.025%	Efcortelan
Cordran cream 0.05%	Fucibet H
Diprosone lotion 0.02%	Hydrocal
Kenalog cream 0.1%	Nystaform HC
Locoid cream 0.1%	Synalar 1:10
Synalar cream 0.025%	Tarcortin
Valisone cream 0.1%	Tynodine
Valisone lotion 0.1%	Vioform HC
Westcort cream 0.2%	
Westcort ointment	
Group VI	
Tridesilon cream 0.05%	
Locorten cream 0.03%	
Synalar solution 0.01%	
Hytone 2.5%	
Dexamethasone	
Elocon	
Group VII	
Hytone I %	
Dexamethasone	
Elocon	

Topical vitamin D treatments

There are several new and effective topical treatments that have become available over the last few years. One of these, a vitamin D3 analogue, calcipotriol or calcipotriene ointment, has been approved in different European countries. Most patients get improvement with calcipotriene and, unlike topical corticosteroids, it does not cause skin thinning or the sudden worsening of psoriasis that sometimes follows the discontinuation of the topical corticosteroid. Some patients develop skin irritancy around the psoriasis areas and the ointment may also produce a skin rash if applied to the face. It is available in cream, ointment and scalp formulations.

Calcitriol, another vitamin D ointment, also improves psoriasis, but it also seems to increase calcium levels in the blood. This is also less effective than calcipotriene.

Dovonex cream and ointment

Dovonex is the trade name for the vitamin D related compound known as calcipotriol in Europe and calcipotriene in the USA.

These creams and ointments are very useful for improving psoriasis. They have a major advantage (together with Tazorac gel) that they do not produce skin thinning or rebound worsening of psoriasis after stopping treatment that can occur with stronger topical cortisones.

Dovonex cream is less messy than Dovonex ointment but also slightly less effective. I will often suggest that patients apply the cream in the morning and the ointment at night.

They are often effective for plaque-like psoriasis. Some patients develop dermatitis on their faces from Dovonex — they should wash their hands after applying Dovonex to their body psoriasis to minimize facial contact.

Dovonex can be combined with other treatments like topical cortisones, phototherapy or systemic treatments (see page 00).

It is also possible to combine Dovonex cream or ointment in the mornings with tazarotene gel at night to thick patches of psoriasis.

Dovonex scalp solution may be useful in mild types of scalp psoriasis but generally is only partly effective for more chronic or severe scalp psoriasis.

Dovonex preparations are a safe and frequently effective way of improving psoriasis.

> **TIPS ON USING DOVONEX CREAM**
>
> - *Apply small amounts of cream or ointment twice daily to psoriasis initially.*
> - *Avoid putting it on your face.*
> - *Wash hands after applying to reduce facial contact.*
> - *Your doctor may give you another cream like a cortisone to apply at another time of day.*

Tazorac gel for psoriasis

Tazorac (known as Zorac in Europe) is the trade name for tazarotene, which is one of a class of drugs called retinoids which are related in structure to vitamin A. These drugs include isotretinoin (Accutane, USA; Ro-Acutane, UK) and acitretin (Soriatane, USA; Neotegison, UK) which are used by mouth for treating more severe acne and psoriasis respectively. When this type of drug is given by mouth (orally) several side-effects are noticed by patients. These side-effects include excessive dryness, chapping and scaling of the skin and lips. Also, problems with liver damage and elevation of blood fat (cholesterol and triglyceride) occur in some patients.

For these reasons topical retinoids would be a significant advantage because these side-effects would not be expected.

1n 1997, Tazorac gel became available in several countries for treating psoriasis. I have been involved in the research and development of this therapy for several years with the pharmaceutical company Allergan. Our first studies involved finding the ideal concentration of this gel. We found two concentrations — 0.1% and 0.05% — to be effective for treating psoriasis.

Following these initial studies, two gel concentrations were studied in hundreds of psoriasis patients. *Figures 13–16* show responses to Tazorac.

We have learned how to treat patients with this gel to optimize the treatment while reducing its side-effects.

Tazorac gel in psoriasis

We found the gel to be effective for mainly the common, plaque type of psoriasis and for scalp psoriasis. Because topical retinoids can cause skin irritancy (itching and burning) it is important to learn how to use it carefully. Here are some guidelines for using tazarotene gel:

Figure 13
(a) Before treatment and (b) 13 weeks after Tazorac 0.1% gel nightly.

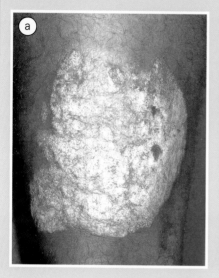
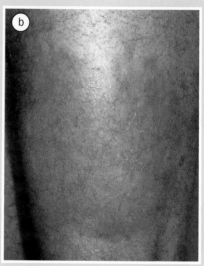

- Only apply the gel at night — allow at least 15 minutes before bed.

- Only apply small amounts of the gel to the psoriasis patches.

- Try to avoid applying the gel to the surrounding skin around the psoriasis.

- You should apply an emollient or moisturizer *before* applying the gel to the psoriasis spots. This will help to reduce drying and redness on the surrounding skin.

- After you have applied the gel wash your hands with water and soap.

- Avoid contact of your eyes, eyelids and mouth with the gel.

- Wait at least 30 minutes after bathing or showering before applying the gel.

- Make sure your skin is dry before applying the gel.

Figure 14
Before (a) and after (b) 6 weeks of Tazorac 0.05% gel. There is only partial improvement at this time. Options include continued treatment with Tazorac 0.1% gel nightly, using a topical cortisone cream (e.g. Elocon) or Dovonex cream/ointments each morning or receiving ultraviolet or careful sun exposure.

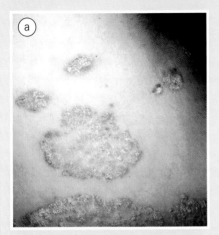
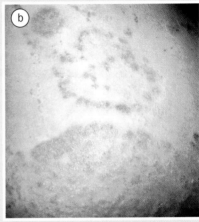

Figure 15
(a) Before treatment and (b) after finishing a course of Tazorac gel nightly.

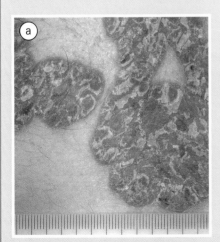
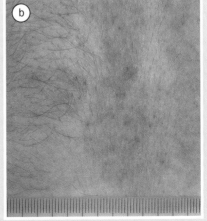

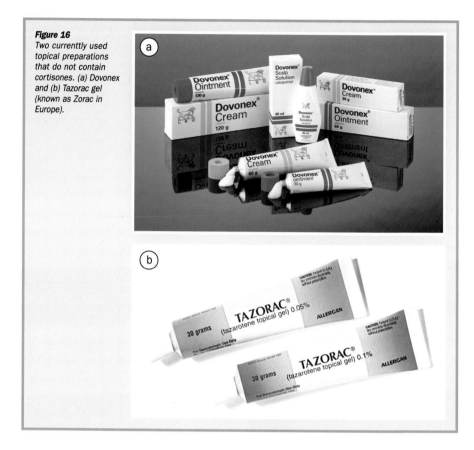

Figure 16
Two currenttly used topical preparations that do not contain cortisones. (a) Dovonex and (b) Tazorac gel (known as Zorac in Europe).

- If your skin becomes dry or irritated from the gel, then temporarily stop the gel until this improves. This may take several days.

- You may be given a prescription for a topical cortisone cream to apply in the morning to the psoriasis.

- You may be advised to receive UVB or sunlight by your doctor. In this case, never apply the gel before the UVB or sunlight — only in the evening *after* the UVB or sunlight. Get clear details from your doctor *before* trying this combination of treatments.

- If you are a fertile woman you must not become pregnant while you are using tazarotene gel. You should ask your doctor about contraception.

Note:
Tazorac gel can occasionally cause a skin reaction that is too severe for that particular patient to continue with this treatment. Sometimes we can interrupt the treatment and go back to it once the skin reaction has cleared.

Tars

Although there are three different types of tars used to treat skin disorders (shale, wood and coal), coal tars seem to be the most effective in controlling psoriasis. Used alone, coal tars are not very effective; but when used in conjunction with ultraviolet therapy, topical corticosteroids and/or with Anthralin spray, they have proven beneficial to combat psoriasis. These combinations of tars and other therapies may be used either on an outpatient or inpatient basis.

One possible treatment plan would call for a patient with localized psoriasis to apply a topical steroid cream or ointment once or twice a day and then apply a tar preparation at night before going to bed. Your doctor will develop a regime that is appropriate for your condition and your schedule.

One annoying problem with tar is its messiness. It can stain both clothing and furnishings, so I recommend applying the tar at least 15 minutes before dressing or going to bed so that the maximum amount of tar will have been absorbed into the skin. Still, it is advisable to wear older clothing or clothing that is already stained when tar has been applied. Many purified tar gels, lotions, creams or oils are less likely to stain clothing after they have been on the skin for several minutes.

Unless your doctor advises you otherwise, avoid exposing coal tar-treated areas of the skin to the sun. Tar treatment increases the risk of sunburn. Of course, if skin infection, redness or stinging of the skin result from using tar preparations, you should suspend your treatment and consult your dermatologist. *Table 2* lists some nonprescription coal tar products. Recently, coal tar-containing shampoos have been subjected to restriction by the US authorities because of perceived fears of increased skin cancer risk.

Keratolytics

These clear, nongreasy lotions, creams or gels help to remove very thick scales and work well in conjunction with other topical treatments, such as tar and/or Anthralin (Dithranol).

Table 2
Tar products.

USA	UK
Aquatar Gel	Alphosyl
Baker's P and S Plus Gel	Balneum
Estar Tar Gel	Clinitar cream
Fototar Tar Cream	Gelcotar
T-Derm Tar Oil	Polytar
T-Derm Tar and Salicylic Acid Scalp Lotion	Psoriderm
	Psorigel
	Psorin

Also available as an alternative to crude coal tar, liquor carbonis detergens (usually between 5 and 20% concentrations in cream, ointment or oils).

- *Many of these products can be messy and stain clothing and furnishings.*
- *Apply small amounts and rub them well into the skin. Use old or stained garments as clothing after applying the coal tars.*
- *Many purified tar gels, lotions, creams or oils will cease staining your clothes after they have been on the skin for several minutes.*
- *Avoid any exposure of coal tar-treated skin to sunlight unless advised by your doctor. He may advise sun or ultraviolet treatments after you apply the coal tar, but these have to be done with his advice to avoid sun burning.*

Also available as additives for bathwater.

Balnetar

Polytar emollient

I usually advise patients to apply a keratolytic agent such as salicylic acid, lactic acid, glyolic acid or ammonium lactate lotion twice a day. Patients who combine this with their tar preparation by mixing the two together in the palm of their hand often see greater results than if they use each agent singly.

Anthralin (Dithranol)

Anthralin (Dithranol) is a synthetic substance made from anthracene, a coal tar derivative. It has been used in the treatment of psoriasis since the nineteenth century. Anthralin (Dithranol) is a relatively safe prescription medication that can be applied as an ointment, paste, cream or stick, and helps to relieve many patients. Anthralin (Dithranol) takes longer to work than steroids, in many cases up to 6 weeks; it can also irritate the skin and some patients cannot tolerate it even in small concentrations. Anthralin has another major drawback: it is sure to stain anything it touches, including normal skin, clothing, tile grout and linoleum. Ceramic shower tiles should rinse clean, if they do not, use a little bleach. Skin staining is actually a sign that the Anthralin is working *(see Figure 17)*. As it does not stain psoriatic skin, the staining means that the skin is clearing up. The skin immediately surrounding the plaque will probably stain, but this should clear up a few weeks after the psoriasis itself has cleared. Stained skin can also be treated with salicylic acid or another keratolytic agent.

Many patients use Anthralin in conjunction with topical steroids, PUVA, oral retinoids and tar-based therapy. Some patients use Anthralin (Dithranol) 'Minutes' or 'short contact' therapy. In this procedure,

Anthralin (Dithranol) cream or ointment is incorporated into an oil-in-water emulsion (Nivea oil or Eucerin, for example). It must be fresh to be effective. Fresh Anthralin (Dithranol) has a bright yellow colour. Once applied, you wash it off between 15 and 60 minutes later with liquid soap and water and an old washcloth. Then lather with a mild soap and finish with a moisturizer.

Anthralin (Dithranol) is applied only to the psoriatic lesions and must be rubbed in well *(see Figures 18 and 19)*. Any excess should be wiped off. Wear plastic disposable gloves or wash your hands carefully after applying the Anthralin. The Anthralin is left in place for increasing periods of time as follows:

• Day 1: 15 minutes (if no irritation occurs).

• Day 2: 30 minutes (if no irritation occurs).

• Day 3: 45 minutes (if no irritation occurs).

After day 4, if no irritation occurs, increase to 60 minutes until clearing occurs and the lesion cannot be fel. *(see Figure 18)*. Do not apply Anthralin (Dithranol) to your face or groin; ask your dermatologist how to treat lesions in those areas. At the end of the contact time, the Anthralin should be thoroughly washed off with soap under running water in the shower.

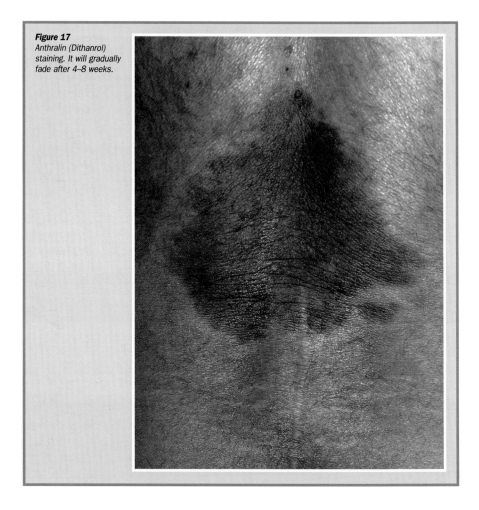

Figure 17
Anthralin (Dithanrol) staining. It will gradually fade after 4–8 weeks.

The following precautions will help reduce or prevent irritation.

- Do not apply Anthralin (Dithranol) to normal skin. Normal skin becomes irritated much faster than psoriatic lesions.

Figure 18
Psoriasis plaque (patches) on elbows. Before (a) and after (b) 8 weeks Anthralin (Dithanrol) 'short contract' treatment for 1 hour each day. (These photographs generously provided by Dr Alan Menter).

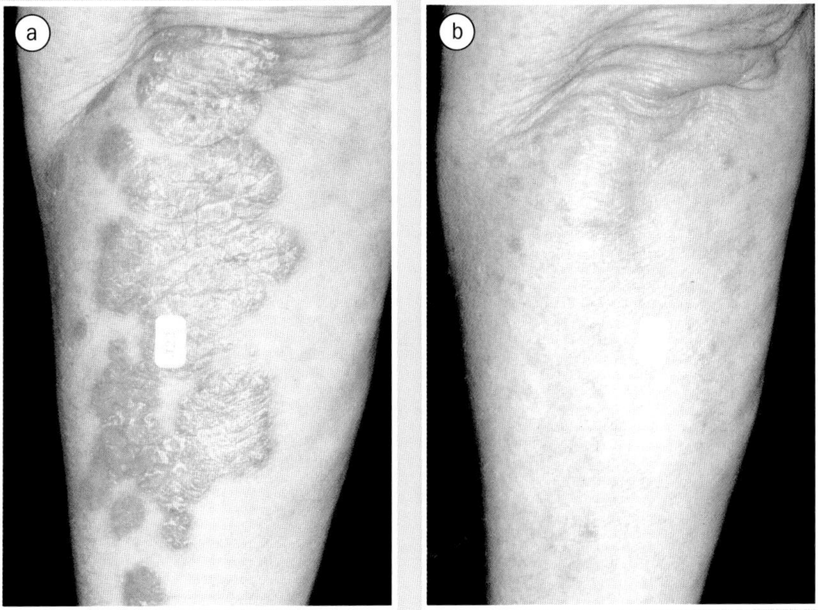

- Cover all Anthralin-treated areas with loose, old clothes while the Anthralin is in place. This will prevent the Anthralin on a lesion on one part of the body from rubbing onto normal skin on another part of the body; for example, from one leg onto the other leg.

- Wash hands carefully after the application and be careful not to touch an Anthralin-treated area and then an untreated area.

- Keep the Anthralin away from eyes. If eye irritation occurs, rinse your eyes thoroughly and call your doctor. If children are present while you are using the Anthralin, extreme caution must be taken to prevent their accidental contact with the Anthralin.

- There are special Dithranol scalp preparations (e.g. Drithoscalp).

- Newer Dithranol preparations such as Micanol may reduce instances of staining of the skin.

Emollients/moisturizers

Particularly valuable in helping patients with dry skin, emollients commonly used in cream or lotion form are an important component of psoriasis therapy. Emollients seem to slow the loss of water through the skin layers that result from frequent bathing and phototherapy and also enhance the effectiveness of phototherapy. Often, patients apply an emollient immediately before phototherapy sessions.

The thicker the cream or lotion, the more effective the emollient is likely to be. Vaseline Pure Petroleum Jelly, for example, is highly effective. It is very important to use emollients after bathing or showering. Most patients are advised to apply moisturizers twice daily and to choose the one they like best to ensure that they are regularly used in order to derive the greatest benefit. You may want to use one that is light for daytime and a heavier, thicker emollient for night-time, when the greasy nature of the emollient won't interfere with your clothing and activities. Scrupulous attention to moisturizing can relieve you of the pain of dry skin and also reduce scaling and inflammation. In addition, moisturizers have no side-effects to worry about. There are dozens of moisturizers available over the counter, including such well-known products as Lubriderm Cream or Moisture Cream or Lotion, Vaseline Dermatology Formula Cream or Lotion, Aquaphor Cream, Eucerin Cream or Lotion, Lac-Hydrin Moisture Lotion, Cetaphil, or Neutrogena Body Oil or Lotion.

EMOLLIENTS/MOISTURIZERS USA

Acid Mantle Creme and Lotion

Alpha Keri Shower and Bath Oil

Aqua Glycolic Hand & Body Lotion

Aquaphor Cream

Carmol 10 Lotion or Carmol 20 Cream

Complex 15 Moisturizing Cream and Lotion

Eucerin Cream (or Lotion)

Lac-Hydrin 5% Lotion

Lac-Hydrin 12% Lotion

Lubriderm Cream (or Lotion)

Lubriderm Lubath Bath Shower Oil

MD Forte Hand & Body Cream

Moisturel Cream

Moisturel Lotion

Neutrogena Norwegian Formula Hand Cream

Neutrogena Facial Moisturizer

Neutrogena Body Oil

Neutrogena Lotion for Hand and Body

Petrolatum White USP

Purpose Dry Skin Cream

Shepherd's Cream Lotion, Skin Cream or Soap

Vaseline Dermatology Formula Cream or Lotion

Vaseline Pure Petroleum Jelly Skin Protectant

UK

Alcoderm Cream/Lotion

Alpha Keri Bath Oil

Aquadrate Cream

Aveeno Bath Oil

Aveeno Cream

Aveeno Oilated/Regular

Balneum Bath Oil

Balneum Plus Bath Oil

Balneum Plus Cream

Caladryl Cream

Caladryl Lotion

Calendolon Ointment

Calmurid Cream

Dermalex

Dermamist

Dermol

Diprobase Cream

Diprobase Ointment

Diprobath

E45 Bath

E45 Cream

E45 Wash

Emulsiderm

Epaderm

Eurax Cream

Eurax Lotion

Hewletts Cream

Humiderm

Hydromol Cream

Hydromol Emollient

Imuderm

Infaderm

Kamillosan Ointment

Keri Therapeutic Lotion

Lacticare

Lipobase

Morhulin

Nupercanial

Nutraplus

Oilatum Cream

Oilatum Emollient

Oilatum Gel

Oilatum Plus

RBC Cream

Sprilon

Sudocream

Ultrabase Cream

Unuentum Merck

Some risks of advertised non-prescription treatments — the Skin Cap deception

Patients with psoriasis are frequently bombarded with advertising and claims for 'psoriasis cures' that make encouraging reading. Some of these have beneficial effects such as products containing coal tars, salicylic acid, alphahydroxyacids and others.

Unfortunately, some of the suppliers of these advertised products make misleading claims and have misled the user as to their real contents.

One such example, recently, was Skin Cap. This was advertised widely in the USA and Europe as containing activated zinc pyrithione and being highly effective for psoriasis. Skin Cap was rapidly effective but the psoriasis quickly returned (often more severely) when the Skin Cap was stopped. The product was investigated and discovered to contain different strong cortisones, which was the reason it was so quickly effective. However, many patients developed cortisone-caused skin thinning and what is known as 'cortisone rebound' (severe worsening of psoriasis). The manufacturers tried to deny the existence of the cortisones. This was a dangerously mislabelled product and highlights the risks of relying on non-prescription advertised treatments at times.

Sunbathing, ultraviolet and PUVA therapy

8

The sun's ultraviolet rays provide the most natural psoriasis treatment available. In fact, nearly 80% of people with psoriasis have observed that their condition improves in sunny climates. Conversely, your psoriasis may worsen in the winter, because of a lack of sunlight — also your mood may change when the days get shorter. Hormonal or biochemical changes that occur in the winter months may also explain exacerbated winter psoriasis, but more research is still needed to confirm this theory.

Before you begin a sun treatment programme, your dermatologist should take a careful history to learn how your skin reacts to sunlight exposure, and determine whether you have any existing skin cancers or have a family history of skin cancer.

People who have had skin cancer in addition to psoriasis must realize that they are at greater risk for developing new skin cancers in any part of the body and should exercise great caution when exposing themselves to the sun's powerful rays. Any areas of the skin that do not have psoriasis, such as the face, should be carefully and consistently protected with sunscreen to avoid any excessive sunlight damage and to reduce the risks of skin cancer and premature aging. Skin cancer patients undergoing sun or ultraviolet therapy should also be examined for new growths at least every 6 months.

Ultraviolet phototherapy

Ultraviolet B (UVB), also known as sunburning ultraviolet, is also known to improve several skin diseases — especially psoriasis. Modern phototherapy has been developed from this knowledge.

Phototherapy is often used for various skin problems — including psoriasis, lichen planus, itching, eczema, mycosis fungoides and some kinds of acne. Treatment involves exposing a patient to artificially generated ultraviolet light for varying lengths of time. UVB phototherapy will not cure your psoriasis, but it can effectively control or improve the disease.

Typically, UVB treatments start with only a few seconds of light exposure and the time is then gradually increased. Clearing or improvement takes an average of 15–20 treatments, after which your skin may stay relatively clear with one treatment every 1–2 weeks. Many patients may then stop treatments. Of course, each patient will vary in the number of treatments per week and the

time it will take to reach clearing, but the 'average' patient initially requires 3 or 4 treatments each week to clear.

Some patients may develop a mild sunburn from the UVB. If this occurs, consult your dermatologist or treatment centre staff. You will not necessarily need to stop the treatment if a sunburn occurs. UVB has several other potential side-effects. Patients often develop a moderate to deep suntan which usually fades within 6–8 weeks after cessation of therapy. Fortunately, few patients complain about this; despite all the dermatologists' warnings, we are still a suntan-worshipping society.

Unfortunately, increased incidence of skin cancer may occur later in some patients who have had many UVB treatments. Because genital skin is particularly susceptible to cancer, patients must protect the groin area during UVB therapy. And, because the light rays can also damage your eyes, you will be required to wear protective eye goggles during your light treatment.

Ultraviolet therapy is best practised in a dermatology treatment centre, but this is sometimes not practical or convenient for patients who live or work too far away. If going to the doctor the 3–5 times a week recommended for 3–6 weeks is inconvenient for you, home ultraviolet therapy may be appropriate. However, many home ultraviolet machines are not powerful enough to clear patients with extensive psoriasis. Patients with more severe disease really need to be treated initially in a professional treatment centre, and then they may control the disease with their home-based unit.

Before beginning this treatment, your dermatologist will want to feel relatively certain that you will improve with this regimen. You need to be instructed carefully in how to administer home ultraviolet treatments, and you must remember that you need full skin examinations at a minimum of every 3 months while conducting home ultraviolet therapy. Even after stopping therapy, you will require annual skin evaluations to ensure that there are no signs of early skin cancer.

UVB can be combined with agents such as acitretin or etretinate *(Figure 19)*.

If administering UVB treatments at home, you must take the following precautions:

- Wear UV protective eyeglasses during treatment.

- Carefully set the machine timer as recommended by the manufacturer to avoid burning reactions.

- Visit your dermatologist every 3 months for routine skin examinations.

PUVA phototherapy

The photosensitizing drug known as psoralen has been used successfully with long wavelength ultraviolet light for the treatment of psoriasiss. The psoralen capsules make the skin sensitive and responsive to the light. Without the psoralen, the light does not treat the skin condition effectively.

One of the first reports of the use of PUVA with oral 8-methoxypsoralen in the treatment of psoriasis was published in 1974. Subsequently, a long-term follow-up study has confirmed the efficacy of PUVA, but questions regarding the long-term risk of skin cancer remain. Recent studies have suggested melanoma skin cancer may occur in a small number of psoriasis patients who have been treated with large amounts of PUVA.

The ultraviolet sources used in PUVA therapy contain broad-spectrum UVA fluorescent bulbs. The higher the intensity of UVA source, the shorter the treatment times required. Many different types of UVA units are available, among them upright cabinets containing 56 or more separate fluorescent tubes. Most units are vertical, but horizontal 'lie-down' units are also available, and are useful for some elderly patients or patients who develop fainting episodes after long periods of standing.

Figure 19
Before (a) and after (b) acitretin and UVB treatment.

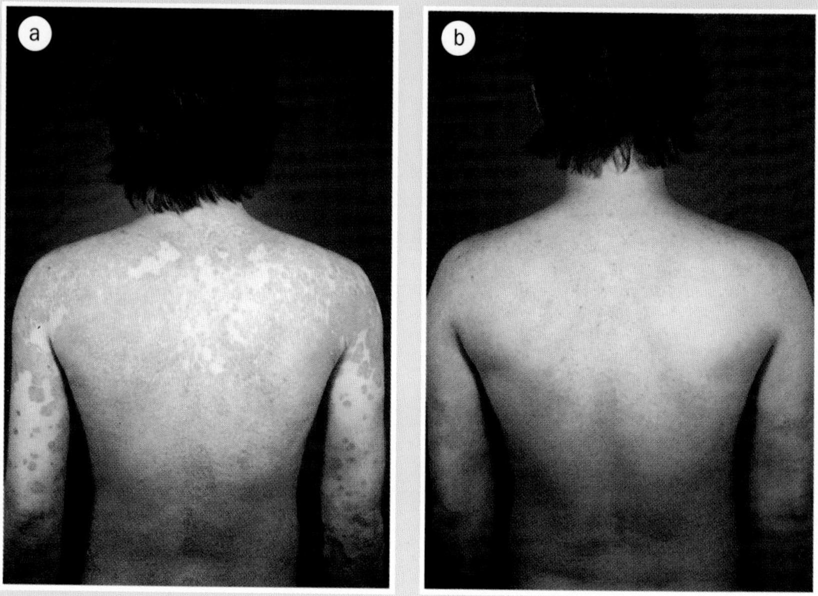

Who is a good PUVA candidate?

Dermatologists select patients for PUVA phototherapy very carefully because of the treatments' potential for long-term skin damage. PUVA phototherapy is only appropriate for those with incapacitating psoriasis, previous failure of conventional topical therapy or of tar and ultraviolet phototherapy, and rapid relapse after the above forms of therapy.

Your doctor will also want to make sure that you don't have any conditions in which PUVA is contraindicated, such as photosensitive diseases, use of photosensitive drugs, previous or present skin cancers, previous X-ray therapy to the skin, or cataracts.

Before you begin your PUVA programme, and every 12 months into the therapy, you will have to undergo an ophthalmological examination to ensure that there are no eye conditions that would preclude your taking part in the photo-treatment programmes. You will use special plastic grey or green sunglasses on the day of the treatment programme and during the light therapy.

Because some of the psoralen stays in the skin for approximately 8 hours after it has been taken, it is important to avoid exposure to sunlight after the treatment. Wear long-sleeved shirts and long trousers and use plenty of sunscreen on unprotected areas.

PUVA has other potential side-effects. Twenty percent of PUVA patients experience nausea and stomach upset from the psoriasis pills. This can often be alleviated by taking pills with food or milk.

Psoralen capsules have not been proven safe during pregnancy, so women are advised to use effective methods of birth control while taking part in this PUVA programme.

Some treatment centres also offer baths containing a psoralen drug. The patient bathes and then immediately receives UVA. This is very useful for patients where the psoralen pills cause nausea and sickness.

A more recent type of psoralen (5-methoxy-psoralen), which produces much less nausea, is now available in Europe and we are currently studying this drug in the USA.

The Dead Sea and Soap Lake: Two natural healing environments

The Dead Sea in Israel is the lowest point on the earth's surface, 1312 feet below sea level. King Herod used to travel to the Dead Sea thousands of years ago to revitalize his spirit and body. People have found this region wonderfully therapeutic, particularly for psoriasis, arthritis and eczema.

What's so special about the Dead Sea? For one thing, the additional layers of the earth's atmosphere there filter out the shorter, more harmful ultraviolet rays while allowing the longer UVA rays to penetrate. As a result, patients can expose their skin to the sun for a long time without burning. The local air is also the richest in oxygen — 10% more than at the Mediterranean Sea level. The air near the Dead Sea also contains a high concentration of bromide, a chemical found in many sedatives.

Some doctors feel that the hydration of the skin by the Dead Sea water, which contains a very high mineral content, may also explain the area's therapeutic quality.

Patients usually remain at the Dead Sea for 4–5 weeks to obtain maximum improvement. Their psoriasis may reappear after they have been home for a while, but ultraviolet therapy, either in the dermatologist's clinic or at home, may stem the re-emergence of the condition.

Those unable to travel to Israel may want to visit the small town of Soap Lake in Central Washington, USA, a popular haven for psoriatics and arthritics. Like the Dead Sea, Soap Lake contains an unusually high mineral content located in a dry desert climate. Lake water is piped into many of the town's motels, and hot mineral baths are also available. For more information, write to:

The Soap Lake Chamber of Commerce, PO Box 433, Soap Lake, WA 98851, USA or call 509 246 1821.

Oral and injectable medications

9

If you have extremely severe or disabling psoriasis, or have disfiguring disease in parts of the body such as hands, nails, scalp and face, your doctor may prescribe oral medications or intramuscular injections. You may hear your dermatologist refer to these as 'systemic' medications or treatments. Make sure that you are fully informed about the possible side-effects of these treatments; then judge for yourself — in consultation with your dermatologist — whether you are willing to take these risks in the hope that the drugs will substantially clear your condition.

There is a wide variety of oral medications, including etretinate (called Tigason in the UK and Tegison in the USA), acitretin (called Psoriatane in the UK and Neotegison in the USA) methotrexate, Cyclosporine, azulfidine, hydroxyurea and Azathioprine.

Etretinate or acitretin

These drugs are frequently referred to as vitamin A derivatives and are also known as retinoids. As retinoids are related to vitamin A, you should avoid taking vitamin A supplements because they may add to the unwanted side-effects of these drugs. Check with your doctor or pharmacist if you have any questions about vitamin supplements.

Etretinate and acitretin have been available over the past decade and have proven to be particularly successful in treating general pustular psoriasis. Patients frequently clear more completely when they have taken retinoids in conjunction with their PUVA or ultraviolet therapy *(Figure 20)* than when they undergo light therapy alone. That is because the retinoid reduces the amount of ultraviolet rays needed for therapy, and the combination improves the efficacy of the treatment as a whole.

Figure 20
Severe psoriasis of the feet. Before (a) and after (b) 8 weeks of oral acitretin. Other successful treatment plans include tazarotene gel and PUVA phototherapy.

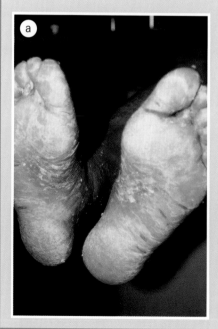
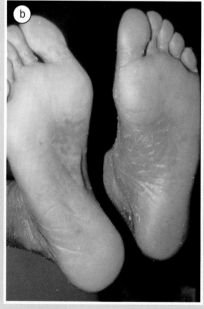

The dosage of etretinate or acitretin varies from patient to patient, with the number of capsules you must take determined specifically for you by your doctor. Periodically during treatment your doctor may change the amount of medicine you need to take. Make sure you follow the schedule you are given. If you miss a dose, do not double the next dose. If you have any questions, call your doctor.

Side-effects of etretinate include dryness of the skin, mouth and lips; hair loss; increased fat levels in the blood; altered liver function and bony overgrowths on the skeleton (this occurs only after prolonged use of the retinoid). Furthermore, etretinate cannot be prescribed for women of child-bearing age because the drug lingers in the body long after it has been ingested and may harm a developing fetus. Fertile women can use Acitretin. It is popularly used for severe acne and is occasionally used in treating general-ized pustular psoriasis. Women should avoid becoming pregnant while taking acitretin and for 2 years after stopping the drug.

Etretinate generally results in improvement in most patients. Some patients, in fact, have obtained complete clearing of their disease after 4–9 months of therapy. You should keep in mind, however, that because some degree of relapse commonly occurs within a few months after therapy is discontinued, most patients require long-term therapy with etretinate. Also, because each patient's dosage regimen may vary, you should discuss your exact course of therapy with your doctor.

Like many patients, you may find that your psoriasis will get worse during the first month of treatment with these drugs. Occasionally patients experience more redness or itching at first, but these symptoms usually subside as treatment continues. Blood tests will be necessary before and during treatment to check your body's response to the drugs.

You may have to wait 2 or 3 months before you realize the full benefit of etretinate. In the first few weeks, perhaps before you see any healing, you may begin to experience some side-effects. You can expect, most often, to find peeling of the fingertips, palms and soles; chapped lips, dry skin and nose; loss of hair; eye irritation; itching; excessive thirst; bone/joint pain; rash; fatigue; red scaly face; sore mouth and skin fragility. If you develop any of these side-effects, check with your doctor to determine if any change in the amount of your medication is needed. Also, ask your doctor to recommend an emollient if drying or chapping develops. If you wear contact lenses, you may find that you are less able to tolerate them during and after therapy. Patients taking etretinate occasionally lose some hair. The extent of hair loss that you may experience and whether or not your hair will return after treatment cannot be determined.

Patients also sometimes experience decreased night vision; since the onset of this problem can be sudden, you should be particularly careful when driving any vehicle at night. If you experience any visual difficulties, stop taking etretinate or acitretin and consult your doctor.

At the time of writing this book, it is understood that etretinate will be withdrawn from the USA and be replaced by acitretin.

Methotrexate

Methotrexate, which has been used for psoriasis treatment longer than any other internal medication, is usually taken once a week either orally or by injection. While very effective, this drug must be used with caution and there are several limitations. Patients must have no history of liver disease or of excessive alcohol consumption. Kidney function must also be normal so that the drug can clear itself easily from the body. Aspirin and arthritis medications could increase the risks of methotrexate toxicity, so consult your dermatologist before taking them. Ideally, patients should see their doctors

every 4 weeks while on methotrexate. If the treatment lasts beyond 12 months, it is important to have a liver biopsy, because methotrexate can cause fibrosis damage to the liver. A liver biopsy is done with a tiny needle inserted through the skin into the liver to extract a small liver sample. The procedure is done under local anaesthetic.

Most side-effects can be detected before they become serious, and your doctor will keep you under close supervision, arranging regular visits and laboratory tests. For the safe treatment of your psoriasis, it is important that you carry out your doctor's instructions faithfully and promptly report any side-effects or symptoms you may develop.

How to take methotrexate

Unlike most medications, methotrexate is given weekly, rather than daily, with the weekly dose taken either as a single or divided dose. If you accidentally take your dose too often, notify your doctor at once. If an accidental overdose occurs, an antidote may be necessary and must be given as early as possible.

The most common side-effects of methotrexate are loss of appetite, nausea (but rarely vomiting), diarrhoea, or sores or ulcers in the mouth. If these or other problems trouble you, or if you should develop any signs of infection or unusual bleeding, notify your doctor promptly and before your next dose of methotrexate is due.

Other medicines you are taking may result in an increase in side-effects or a decrease in the effectiveness of methotrexate. Tell your doctor about all the medicines you are taking, whether they are prescription or nonprescription medicines. Do not begin or change the dosage of any medicine without first checking with your doctor. This is especially true of aspirin, aspirin-like drugs (the so-called nonsteroidal anti-inflammatory drugs), and antibiotics that contain the drug trimethoprim.

Unrelated medical conditions, especially dehydration, can also increase the risk of methotrexate toxicity. Abdominal upset, when accompanied by significant vomiting, diarrhoea, or decreased fluid intake, can lead to dehydration. Notify your doctor if these symptoms develop.

Alcoholic beverages (including beer and wine) may increase some of the side-effects, including the chance of liver damage, and should be severely restricted or avoided altogether.

Side-effects can occur at any time during your treatment. Periodic laboratory tests and sometimes other types of tests arranged by your doctor are necessary for the safe use of methotrexate.

Methotrexate is known to cause birth defects and may cause miscarriage or stillbirth, especially in the first 3 months of pregnancy. Pregnant women must not take methotrexate, and women of childbearing age must not become pregnant while taking the medication. Adequate contraceptive measures are necessary during therapy and for several months thereafter. Consult your doctor before considering pregnancy.

Long-term therapy may result in scarring (fibrosis or cirrhosis) in the liver. At times it may be necessary to have a liver biopsy to determine whether scarring is present. Whether and when to do a liver biopsy is a matter of discussion between you and your doctor.

In addition, very rarely in psoriasis patients, methotrexate can cause a lung reaction similar to pneumonia. The symptoms are usually fever, cough (often dry and hacking) and shortness of breath (which can become severe).

Cyclosporine

Initially used as an immune suppressive drug in organ transplant patients, Cyclosporine has been found to work very well and very rapidly in treating severe psoriasis and psoriatic arthritis *(Figure 21)*. As with methotrexate, it is best not to use Cyclosporine over prolonged periods of time because the drug suppresses the body's immune system. Protracted use theoretically may lead to increased risks of cancer particularly lymphoma, although a higher cancer risk has not been seen yet in psoriasis patients treated with Cyclosporine.

As a further precaution, Cyclosporine should be taken only by patients with normal blood pressure and kidney function. Given the powerful nature of the drug, only a dermatologist experienced in its use should prescribe it.

Figure 21
A patient with severe psoriasis. Before (a) and after (b) 12 weeks of Cyclosporine by mouth. Notice the increase in body hair growth on Cyclosporine treatment. This can occasionally be a problem for patients – particularly women.

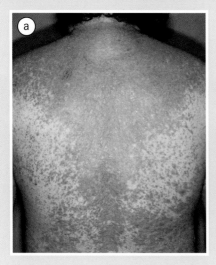 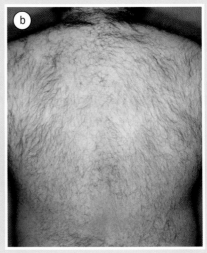

Typically, Cyclosporine is used to bring about a remission of psoriasis and maintenance therapy is continued with another treatment such as UVB or UVA and/or methotrexate or acitretin. In some cases, however, maintenance therapy may be continued with low dose Cyclosporine. Additionally, because each patient's dosage regimen may vary, you should discuss your exact course or therapy with your doctor.

As with all systemic treatments, Cyclosporine does have potential side-effects. A temporary reduction in kidney function, which can be detected by laboratory tests, sometimes occurs with Cyclosporine. The drug has also been associated with permanent kidney damage. Kidney functions will be monitored by blood and urine tests throughout the treatment and Cyclosporine will be stopped if any significant changes occur.

Another risk is the development of lymphoma (cancer of the lymph glands) in patients who have received high doses of Cyclosporine, especially if they took other medications such as cortisone-like steroids. Therefore, you must not take any other immunosuppressants such as steroids while taking Cyclosporine. The doses of Cyclosporine you will be taking are lower than those given to transplant patients. It is not known if the risks of Cyclosporine causing lymphoma at these lower dosages are

less; it is expected that they will be, but there is no current clinical proof.

Various forms of cancer (bladder, lung, breast and cervical cancer) have been observed in patients using Cyclosporine to treat psoriasis and other diseases.

Other potential side-effects of Cyclosporine include: high blood pressure, increased hair growth, enlargement of the gums, headache, pain in the joints, tiredness, tingling in the fingers and toes, and shakiness. These side-effects are usually associated with high doses of Cyclosporine and are reversible upon stopping or lowering the dose. Be sure to let your doctor know as soon as possible if you experience any of these side-effects.

You must not take any nonsteroidal anti-inflammatory drugs such as aspirin, Advil or Motrin while taking Cyclosporine. Also you must not take medicines known to interact with Cyclosporine such as:

- Ketoconazole

- Erythromycin

- Phenytoin

- Barbiturates

- Carbamazepine

- Isoniazid

- Rifampicin

After the psoriasis has improved, patients are advised to switch to an alternate type of treatment. There are a number of other internal treatments for severe psoriasis. Hydroxyurea is an old-style anti-cancer drug which is sometimes mildly effective. Combining hydroxyurea with etretinate or acitretin can boost its effectiveness. Blood counts should be monitored carefully while on this medication.

Azathioprine (also known as Immuran) is also an immune-suppressive drug, but not as powerful as Cyclosporine. Although not as effective as etretinate, methotrexate or Cyclosporine, Azathioprine is occasionally used for patients with arthritis and severe skin psoriasis.

Dermatologists may sometimes prescribe other drugs such as the anti-cancer drugs fluorouracil and 6 thioguanine, which can be used on a short-term basis. Cyclosporine is a very potent drug requiring frequent follow-up appointments and blood tests. Be sure to return to your doctor as scheduled. If you have any questions at any point during your treatment, be sure to ask your doctor.

Systemic steroids

Too often, I have seen patients develop severe pustular and exfoliative reactions with their psoriasis when these systemic steroids have been discontinued. Some of the more common types of systemic steroids are prednisone (an oral medication) and triam-cinolone (an intramuscular injection).

Future hopes for finding a cure

10

While we do not yet know the cause of psoriasis, we do know much more today than we did a decade ago. Over the last 10 years, scientists have discovered many of the skin changes now known to produce psoriasis. Among the most important recent discoveries are:

- Biochemical changes that may lead to the thickened skin and abnormal scale in psoriasis. This knowledge has led to new treatments that reduce this thickened skin and scale. It has already led to the development of several new topical drugs that are being tested on patients. Some of these new treatments look very promising.

- Biochemical changes in the psoriastic skin that may cause or be part of the redness or inflammation. Understanding these changes has helped scientists to develop new topical drugs (steroids and nonsteroidals) that have been made more effective in treating psoriasis. Some newer non-steroidal agents may result in further improved treatments with fewer side-effects for psoriasis skin.

• Immune changes that may produce the inflammation abnormalities mentioned above. Understanding these has already allowed an oral drug (Cyclosporine) to be extensively researched in patients with severe psoriasis.

These are exciting and hopeful times for medical research concerning psoriasis. New treatments are being discovered, existing treatments are being improved, future understanding about abnormalities in psoriasis will lead to new treatment approaches and hopefully control or clear the disease.

There are many treatments for psoriasis. The following are just a few of the new therapies that are bringing hope to so many patients:

Topical retinoids

Topical retinoids have been highly effective for a number of different skin diseases, including acne and ichthyoses, and in the treatment of photo-aged skin. Several years ago, retinoic acid was also proven to be effective in treating psoriasis.

The main disadvantage of retinoic acid therapy in psoriasis is skin irritation. As a result, a search for retinoid analogues has resulted in agents that have retained a retinoid-like effect with less skin irritation. Recent studies with a topical acetylenic retinoid have shown this agent to be effective in treating psoriasis. This is now available in several countries and is known as Tazorac (tazarotene gel) in the USA and Canada and Zorac in Europe

Newer vitamin D agents

These may prove to be more effective than calcipotinol, have good safety and are being studied.

Nonsteroidal anti-inflammatory agents

We continue to search for effective topical nonsteroidal anti-inflammatory agents to treat psoriasis. Nonsteroidal anti-inflammatory agents may have advantages over topical corticosteroids in that they are unlikely to cause skin atrophy. Newer agents under investigation show potential efficacy in the treatment of psoriasis in preliminary studies.

New trends in therapy of more severe psoriasis

Recent trends in phototherapy have been designed to improve the efficacy of phototherapy and reduce toxicity. A drug called 8-MOP, dissolved in bathwater, is extremely valuable for patients who develop significant nausea from taking 8-MOP orally. Oral 5-methoxypsoralen (5-MOP) is as effective as 8-MOP PUVA, but appears to have a much lower risk of the acute toxicity problems of nausea.

Use of 'targeted' immune suppressors that reduce inflammation, while having less risk than Cyclosporine, are being researched.

There is hope that over the next few years we will make even greater strides toward curing psoriasis. Perhaps the most exciting research area for the future is the study of the gene or genes that, when inherited, may lead to psoriasis. In the USA, the National Psoriasis Foundation has provided funds to help with this research, which will investigate families who have several members with psoriasis. Similar gene research is being conducted in Europe.

Recent research has shown that when animals have a gene added that is linked with a type of psoriasis arthritis, those animals develop the same disease that occurs in humans. Researchers have known for many years that psoriasis runs in families. More recent research has linked parts of chromosomes (the parts of the body cells that carry the genes) for psoriasis. Newer research techniques have made it possible to continue the search for abnormal or defective genes that are linked with psoriasis.

Time and more research are needed to isolate these abnormal genes. Once the abnormal gene or genes have been found, it will be necessary to determine how and why they do not work normally and what specific abnormality results. If this abnormality can be identified, researchers may be able to design treatments to correct it, and hopefully control psoriasis or even eradicate it.

Case studies

Case study 1: Anthony

Anthony was a 35-year-old patient who had had psoriasis for 20 years. His psoriasis mainly affected his arms and legs, with very stubborn patches on his elbows and knees.

Over the years, he had been treated with cortisone creams and ointments, with temporary relief. The psoriasis would often worsen rapidly after stopping these creams. When he treated himself with coal tar ointment he only found partial improvement. His psoriasis always improved in the summer months and worsened in the winter. Dovonex cream again gave partial improvement.

I decided to treat him with tazarotene gel at night and, for the first 3 weeks, a cortisone cream (Elocon) each morning. This reduced the risk of dermatitis from the tazarotene gel.

After 3 weeks he was improving and I advised him to stop using his Elocon cream. He continued to apply the Tazorac gel at night and has much improved. He now applies moisturizing lotions each morning to his arms and legs. He only applies Tazorac gel when he sees any psoriasis patches reappearing.

Case study 2: Lillian

Lillian is an administrative secretary who developed very severe psoriasis and I was contacted by her employer (with her permission), giving some details about her situation and explaining the need for her to attend my clinic to discuss therapy.

I elected to treat her with coal tar and ultraviolet therapy. Like other patients undergoing this therapy, Lillian came to the treatment centre each day and stayed a minimum of 3 hours. When she arrived at the treatment centre a nurse examined her and then applied special creams and ointments, each containing different concentrations of coal tar, over the entire surface of her affected skin. (These preparations are very messy, but can be used easily in a treatment centre setting.) Lillian wore a special gown provided by the centre to keep the cream and ointments in place. After 2 hours of being covered with the ointments Lillian showered and was then treated with carefully measured amounts of ultraviolet radiation in an ultraviolet cabinet. This combination-style treatment, known as the Goeckerman treatment or Modified

Goeckerman therapy (after the dermatologist who devised it), has been used since the 1920s and is very effective.

Less than 1 month after beginning her daily treatments at the centre, Lillian's skin lesions were 90% cleared! At this point, she went back to work full-time. For another 6 weeks, Lillian came to the treatment centre twice a week to receive an ultraviolet treatment lasting 10 minutes.

Since we stopped the treatments, Lillian has remained clear of any psoriasis. I explained to her that she may experience a recurrence, but if that happens, she knows to come to my office immediately to stop the disease from spreading. Lillian has also been given a supply of oral antibiotics to combat any threat of infection from future sore throats. It is precisely this kind of infection that produced the severe type of guttate psoriasis she suffered.

Case study 3: Bill

Bill is a 35-year-old advertising executive who first developed psoriasis when he was 15. Fortunately, Bill's psoriasis is confined to local scaling red patches on the elbows and on the scalp. The patches on his scalp initially looked like dandruff, with scale and flakes showing on Bill's dark business suits. He was able to control the scalp scaling with the use of tar shampoos that he bought from the pharmacist. However, his scalp became resistant to this shampoo treatment over time, and the patches on his elbows began to thicken.

Bill's main problem was the impact the scalp disease had on his work. Although his colleagues never commented on it, he knew they had all noticed his strange skin disease. Some of them started shying away from him, and he could see the questions in their eyes: Did he have a fungus? Could he have AIDS?

As Bill became estranged from his co-workers, he lost a lot of his confidence. He turned to his family practitioner, who prescribed a variety of cortisone lotions for Bill to use on the scalp twice a day. Unfortunately, many of these lotions made his hair messy and greasy, and while they worked initially, the scalp disease became resistant to their effects.

Bill eventually heard about my treatment centre from a friend who also had psoriasis. After examining him, I offered Bill a choice of treatment options. We began by trying local treatments to control his psoriasis. (I did not want to start him immediately on internal medications because of their side-effects.) I selected a treatment using Anthralin — an old-fashioned treatment used since the late 1800s and by far the most common topical treatment for psoriasis in Europe.

Bill's elbow patches responded well to the Anthralin; but while that was a nice bonus, Bill's first priority was curing the scalp psoriasis. After nurses at the treatment centre instructed Bill carefully in the use of the Anthralin scalp preparation, he began applying the liquid cream to his scalp every evening, keeping it on for increasing amounts of time, starting at 10 minutes and gradually working up to sessions of 1 hour or more. He shampooed the Anthralin off with tar shampoos containing salicylic acid. Over the next 6 weeks, Bill's scalp problem gradually improved, and he was able to reduce the frequency of the Anthralin scalp cream to once or twice a week.

Today, Bill still uses a tar shampoo every day. While it is likely that there will be times in the future when he will require more frequent treatments, Bill is greatly relieved by his progress to date. His relationships with colleagues have mended as well, so that the psoriasis no longer interferes with his work. Best of all, Bill has the secure knowledge that help is available should new outbreaks of his scalp disease occur.

Case study 4: Patrick

Patrick was a healthy, slightly overweight 20-year-old with a family history of psoriasis; both a brother and an uncle suffered from the disease. He developed psoriasis over most of his body after an initial patch appeared on his lower back, but he was able to cope with the familiar (and familial) disease until he developed a puzzling swelling and pain in his finger joints. This was the first sign that Patrick was developing arthritis as part of his psoriasis.

Only about 10% of psoriasis sufferers are afflicted by arthritis, but when psoriatic arthritis strikes, it can become very severe and disabling. Patrick became progressively immobilized by his dual diseases. His arthritis seemed to affect every joint, including his back. Because his knees and his shoulders were swollen and painful, his movement and activity level ground to a halt, and he was confined to bed for weeks at a time. Depressed and bored, Patrick ate to excess, put on weight, and was unable to continue with school or work because of his disabilities.

Patrick was referred to both a dermatologist and rheumatologist (arthritis expert). They initially treated him with arthritis medicine called Indocin, which had little impact on the arthritis, and may have even aggravated his skin problems. He was then treated with a drug called methotrexate which did, initially, help. However, 6 months after treatment began, Patrick's doctors discovered that he had suffered liver damage as a result of the methotrexate and discontinued that therapy. At that point, Patrick almost despaired of receiving effective treatment.

Fortunately, Patrick was referred to a psoriasis specialist who gave him Cyclosporine, which had shown great promise in Europe, and was then being investigated in the USA. Cyclosporine has been used since 1985 to combat the body's instinct to reject transplanted organs. Its application for psoriasis was discovered when two patients with psoriasis had organ transplants and were treated with it. Not only did Cyclosporine control the organ rejection, but it also dramatically improved their psoriasis.

Patrick took his Cyclosporine as a liquid dissolved in orange juice once in the morning and again in the evening. Over the next 3 weeks his psoriasis markedly improved. He soon became more mobile, was able to walk again and even began attending physical therapy sessions to exercise.

Patrick continues to come to the clinic every 4 weeks so that the staff can monitor his blood pressure, which up to now has been very well controlled. Once bedridden and despondent, Patrick is now optimistically considering his future career choices.

Case study 5: Ted

Ted is a retired hardware store owner. When he was 69 years old, he developed scaling patches on his back and elbows, which his family doctor correctly diagnosed as psoriasis. Initially, local cortisone creams and ointments controlled the condition; but then Ted's wife died, tragically and unexpectedly. He was devastated by his loss and began to drink heavily. About 4 months later, Ted's psoriasis began to spread and worsen. A friend recommended one of the local psoriasis support groups of the National Psoriasis Foundation. (See the Appendix for further information about this foundation.) In turn, several members of the support group suggested that Ted see a psoriasis specialist.

By then, nearly 45% of Ted's skin was covered by the red scaling patches of psoriasis, many of them itchy and painful where they cracked.

In discussing different treatment options, Ted said he really did not want to come into the hospital or spend long periods at the treatment centre. He still liked to go into his hardware store part-time and make sure that everything was running smoothly.

As Ted was clearly still emotionally distraught, the dermatologist suggested that he see a psychiatrist in conjunction with his psoriasis treatment. The state of the skin and the psyche are frequently linked, and in Ted's case, it almost certainly was a combination of his wife's death and his psoriasis that caused his emotional distress.

Ted started a treatment programme using PUVA (psoralen UVA phototherapy) at my treatment centre and saw a counsellor about his recent bereavement and the stress induced by his psoriasis. We hoped this plan would help Ted break the cycle of depression and psoriasis by attacking it from both sides.

Unfortunately, Ted became tired and nauseated about 1 hour after taking the psoralen pills that were required for his PUVA therapy (see **Chapter 8** for further details on PUVA treatment). So at a follow-up visit, I instructed Ted to begin dissolving his medication in the bathwater instead of taking it in pill form; my research on PUVA treatment at that time suggested that this might remedy the side-effects.

Ted came to the treatment centre three times a week for his 30-minute psoralen bath, followed immediately by 15 minutes in the UVA light. His psoriasis steadily improved on this regimen, and after 6 weeks I reduced his treatment to twice a week. Four weeks later, Ted was able to cut back to only one treatment a week.

Today, Ted maintains his weekly visits, which are sufficient to control his psoriasis. He may even be able to stop his PUVA therapy if he continues to improve. Many patients do remain clear after several months of the treatment. The psychological counselling has also proved beneficial. With more knowledge of his disease, Ted is better able to cope with the emotional disturbances psoriasis can cause and he has become more outgoing and socially involved.

Case study 6: Sandra

Sandra was an 18-year-old high school student whose cousin had psoriasis. Sandra developed a sore throat that became very severe. Within 2 weeks of that sore throat she developed large numbers of flat, red, slightly scaly patches on the trunk and chest. Her family

practitioner was unsure of the nature of the skin disease and she was referred to our dermatology centre.

It was clear on taking her history and examining Sandra that she was suffering from a condition called guttate psoriasis. This frequently follows a 'strep' or streptococcal sore throat.

We treated Sandra with the oral antibiotic erythromycin for her sore throat and with ultraviolet therapy three times per week. This resulted in significant improvement and clearance of her guttate psoriasis. Sandra has remained psoriasis-free for 2 years now, although it is possible that she may get psoriasis in the future. In addition, if she gets any further sore throats she must immediately start taking her erythromycin antibiotic in an attempt to stop the occurrence of further guttate psoriasis.

Case study 7: Stanley

Stanley was a 35-year-old patient who was referred to the dermatology centre because of gradually worsening thick scaling patches on his elbows and scalp. His scalp scaling became so severe that his scalp felt as though it was enclosed in armour-plated casing.

Because he had previously undergone multiple topical treatments for his scalp psoriasis, I decided to put Stanley on a low dosage of an oral medicine called etretinate. This is a vitamin A-type derivative which can thin the thickened patches of scale in psoriasis. When the scale is thinned by this drug it can allow topical preparations such as the cortisone lotions and Anthralin scalp preparations to work much more efficiently.

Stanley still has his scalp psoriasis, but it has improved sufficiently, and his outlook has also improved. He is able to cope much more adequately with his disease.

Case study 8: Peter

Peter is a 20-year-old carpenter who developed scaling psoriasis patches on the knees and elbows. He also developed nail problems with his psoriasis and within 6 months started to develop arthritis in his fingers and toes. His psoriasis steadily worsened, despite topical treatment from his dermatologist. Peter was put on Indocin and other oral arthritis medicines. Unfortunately, his disease gradually worsened so that he was unable to work because of his psoriasis of the nails, which became very painful, and because of the arthritis in his hands.

I decided, after careful history taking and discussion with Peter, that it was extremely important for him to be able to go back to work as soon as possible, and prescribed a drug called methotrexate, an anti-cancer drug that is used in psoriasis in very low dosages (usually between two and eight pills once or twice a week). It is very effective when there is plaque psoriasis and associated arthritis, as in Peter's case.

Because methotrexate can affect the liver, I decided that it was necessary to see Peter every 4 weeks to repeat careful examination and to make sure that his blood tests were normal. It was also important to make sure that Peter did not drink alcohol or take any other medications for his psoriasis that might interfere with the methotrexate. These included large amounts of aspirins or other arthritis medication.

Peter is now back at work. He still has mild nail psoriasis, but this has not been nearly as painful since starting his methotrexate. Peter is very pleased with his progress to date and I plan to keep him on methotrexate, providing that his blood tests stay normal and his liver biopsy is satisfactory.

Case study 9: Fred

Fred is a 30-year-old research scientist who developed patches of psoriasis when he was a teenager. These became very persistent and always collected on his arms and legs. Although there were only about four patches, Fred was always embarrassed about them — especially around the women he was dating. Routine topical treatments such as topical cortisones did not clear Fred's patches, and Anthralin made the redness and inflammation much worse.

Serendipitously, Fred was planning to attend a scientific meeting in London. While there, I recommended that he use calcipotriol (Dovonex) ointment. This vitamin D analogue has been available in the USA from 1993 and is proving useful for many patients.

Calcipotriol ointment (calcipotriene, as it is known in the USA) enables patients to improve and control their psoriasis. It does not lead to skin thinning as with cortisone creams, nor does it stain the skin like coal tars or Anthralin. Fred has been applying it for 12 months and has already seen a very significant improvement in his psoriasis — he is now only needing the Dovonex for very small patches of skin. We plan to continue this treatment on an 'as needed' basis.

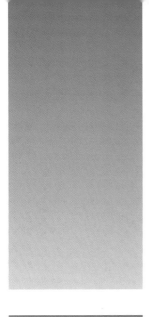

Questions and answers about psoriasis

Many of my patients have lots of questions about psoriasis. Here are some of the most common questions and their answers.

Q: *Is psoriasis infectious or contagious?*

A: Psoriasis is not infectious or contagious. You cannot infect others with it or contract it from other psoriasis sufferers. This is an important point that has to be reiterated frequently to family, friends and employers, who often worry needlessly. A dermatologist should be willing to provide a letter confirming this lack of infectiousness.

Q: *Is psoriasis due to nerves, stress or other emotional factors?*

A: Psoriasis is not caused by stress, but anxiety can and does aggravate the condition. Frequently, several weeks or months pass after an especially stressful period before the psoriasis begins to worsen. Work-related stress, marital conflict and bereavement certainly can contribute to this problem. I once saw an example of this with a patient who had been under severe stress at work. His boss continually pressured him with unrealistic expectations and unfair deadlines. During a particularly pressure-filled period his psoriasis became much more severe with much larger areas of skin affected by psoriasis plaques. The patient left his job to look for another one. His psoriasis grew even worse during this brief period of job hunting. Finally, when he settled into a new and more reasonable work environment, his psoriasis gradually improved and he needed fewer and fewer treatments.

Q: *Can diet improve my psoriasis?*

A: Many patients ask whether their unhealthy diets have caused their psoriasis or whether a particular diet can help alleviate their psoriasis. Diet is of course very important for the maintenance of good health, but it is unlikely to benefit psoriasis directly. However, it is known that diets containing high amounts of omega-3 polyunsaturated fats, such as fish oils, may help to reduce the inflammation caused not only by psoriasis but also by psoriatic arthritis. Omega-3 polyunsaturated fats are especially plentiful in salmon, herring, mackerel and other oily fish. (People who prefer to avoid these fatty fish could take fish oil capsules instead, which may produce the same effect.) A

few of my patients have found that omitting pork from their diets has also helped.

Q: *I have a springtime allergy to grasses. My allergist suggested allergy injection treatments until I told him that I had psoriasis. Can these allergy treatments aggravate my mild case of psoriasis?*

A: It is unlikely that injections that are intended to reduce your response to grass allergy will worsen your psoriasis. These injections generally are very small amounts of the allergic substance and are intended to produce a greater tolerance to the specific allergy. One of the treatments to avoid for severe allergies would be either intramuscular or systemic corticosteroid drugs, e.g. prednisone or triamcinolone. These may temporarily improve your psoriasis, but subsequently your psoriasis may significantly worsen.

Q: *One day I decided to use the raw yolk of an egg on my psoriasis lesions. The itching stopped almost immediately and the scales are disappearing, so I have continued my egg treatments. What makes an egg yolk do this? Will there be any side-effects?*

A: No one can say for sure what agent is likely to have produced the improvement in your psoriasis. Egg yolk contains large amounts of cholesterol and other lipids (fats). It is conceivable that the egg yolk was acting as a moisturizer and it is well known that moisturizers help to reduce the scale accumulation in psoriasis and other skin diseases. The most likely reason therefore is one of the effect of the lipid (fat) content of the egg yolk on your scales.

Q: *What side-effects does methotrexate have on your liver?*

A: Methotrexate is a very effective drug for severe psoriasis and psoriatic arthritis. It can be used orally or by intramuscular or intralesional injections. It is very important for any doctor prescribing methotrexate to question you carefully about the possibility of liver disease. See **Chapter 9** for more information about this drug.

Q: *I was diagnosed with psoriatic pubic symphysitis, an arthritis in the pelvic area that is extremely painful to me. Is there a particular treatment for this type of psoriatic arthritis? Is it common for psoriatic arthritis to occur in a man's pelvis?*

A: Psoriatic arthritis can occur in any joint. While it is most common in the finger and toe joints, it can occur in the rib joints, between the ribs and in the pubic area. The routine treatments for psoriatic arthritis in any area include the use of a variety of nonsteroidal anti-inflammatory agents such as indomethacin, clinoral, voltarin, etc. These drugs would be the first line of treatment. In patients with more severe and persistent arthritis, other agents that might be used include azulfidine, gold or methotrexate in low dosages. Seek the advice of both a dermatologist and a rheumatologist (joint arthritis expert) for your problem.

Q: *My son is 12 years old and has had psoriasis since the age of 4. My good news is that all of a sudden his psoriasis has improved 90%. He has not been on any oral medication except Naproxen for psoriatic arthritis and no topical cream except for moisturizing lotions. Could the varying hormone levels caused by puberty have an effect on the psoriasis? My son hates to admit how improved his psoriasis is because he's afraid it will get worse again.*

A: One of the great puzzles of psoriasis is what initiates spontaneous improvement in so many patients. It is very possible that a change in hormone pattern before puberty can influence psoriasis. We know, for example, that pregnant women often see changes in the severity of their psoriasis.

It is very understandable that your son is afraid that his psoriasis will get worse again. Careful emotional support and reassurance should be given including the reassurance that there are numerous treatments available for psoriasis at the present time.

Q: *What are Nystatin and Amphotericin B cream? I have heard these mentioned as possible treatments for psoriasis and I was wondering if they could help me.*

A: Nystatin is an agent that is effective against yeast infections including Candida. Some researchers have suggested that there is a link between Candida and psoriasis. These agents work in some patients particularly in the skin-fold areas and the head areas such as the scalp.

Amphotericin B cream, produced in France, is not the most effective treatment. I would recommend the ketoconazole shampoo or broad-spectrum imidazole creams (Spectazole, Oxystat, Nizoral, Micatin) instead.

Q: *Do types of psoriasis change in an individual? For instance, I have plaque psoriasis now, but sometimes it changes to guttate, and later on, to pustular. How common are these changes?*

A: Some patients do have changing psoriasis during their lives and a number of different factors can change the pattern of psoriasis. For example, streptococcal sore throats can produce a change of stable plaque psoriasis to guttate psoriasis. The excessive use of stronger topical corticosteroids for long periods or systemic steroids can occasionally produce changes to pustular psoriasis.

Certain medications, such as lithium, can change stable plaque psoriasis to pustular or severe exfoliative psoriasis. In many patients who have frequent changes to more severe pustular psoriasis, it is wise to try and treat the patients with anti-psoriasis treatments that will attempt to stabilize their disease. (For example, if somebody is having recurrent pustular psoriasis they can take low dosage systemic retinoids; if somebody is having recurrent guttate psoriasis then low dosage antibiotics such as erythromycin with frequent throat cultures and appropriate change to an alternative antibiotic are sometimes helpful.)

Q: *Can skin that has been damaged by occlusive use of steroid creams be restored?*

A: This depends on the degree of damage. Sometimes if the skin has been severely thinned by the steroids, it will not recover. However, if the damage has been mild, stopping the corticosteroid or reducing the dosage to a much lower strength can help in skin recovery. There is additional research being conducted with agents such as topical retinoic acid to see if that restores the steroid-induced skin thinning more rapidly.

This is one of the reasons why great care needs to be taken with the use of topical steroids, particularly the strong ones used in the skin-fold areas.

Q: *Do animals get psoriasis, or is it only a human disease?*

A: In fact there have been at least two reports of psoriasis or psoriasis-like conditions developing in rhesus monkeys. In addition, there are now genetically changed rats that have one of the genes added experimentally for psoriatic arthritis (the gene for HLA 27) that have been shown to develop a psoriasis-like condition. Further research in this area is extremely important and may lead to a greater understanding of the causes and the genetic control of psoriasis.

Q: *Why does my psoriasis get worse in the winter and better in the summer?*

A: We are not sure whether this common effect is a direct result of the amount of ultraviolet light available from the summer sun or whether it relates to the length of day. There are various theories about hormonal changes as well as a direct affect of ultraviolet light. While there is still a need for further research, the knowledge that psoriasis improves in the summer has led to the use of ultraviolet phototherapy with artificial sun-lamps in psoriasis. However, too much sunlight or artificial sunlight (ultraviolet) can lead to an increased risk of skin cancer, so it is important to consult your dermatologist for guidelines.

Q: *What factors can make my psoriasis worse?*

A: Several things are known to make psoriasis worse. These include medications such as beta-blockers, lithium and antimalarial drugs as well as some anti-arthritis medications. A common factor in aggravating psoriasis, particularly in teenagers and younger adults, is streptococcal sore throat. This may result in a type of psoriasis called guttate (very small patches) psoriasis. If you get 'strep' throat, begin taking an antibiotic (either erythromycin or penicillin). Your doctor can prescribe these for you and if you are highly susceptible to sore throats, you may want to keep some on hand at all times. Some doctors may not be aware of the link between strepto-coccal sore throat and psoriasis, so it is important that you inform your doctor of your concerns about this.

Another thing that can produce psoriasis in about 30% of patients is skin damage. If you burn, cut or scrape the skin, psoria-sis may occur in that part of damaged skin. This is known as Koebner's phe-nomenon. It is very important for any-body with psoriasis to carefully avoid skin damage, for example, abrasions, burns etc.

Nail psoriasis can also be made worse by a Koebner-type reaction, so do not scrape or clean under the nails or damage the nail in any way. If you are going to be working in the garden or at a manual job, use gloves to protect the nails as much as possible and reduce the risk of further nail damage with psoriasis.

Q: *What do the terms 'steroids' and 'cortisones' mean? Are these dangerous for psoriasis patients?*

A: Cortisones and steroids are common names for treatments used for a variety of diseases. Cortisones are mainly used for the treatment of inflammatory diseases. The steroids or cortisones that are used for skin diseases are not related to the anabolic cortisones or anabolic steroids that are used (and misused) by some athletes for muscle building.

Psoriasis patients should avoid systemic (intramuscular or oral) cortisones wherever possible. (There are a few exceptions, such as patients with severe arthritis or other diseases such as severe asthma that may occasionally need these drugs.) These drugs may drastically worsen the psoriasis in ways that we do not understand. After taking these internal or systemic corti-sones, the psoriasis can become extremely severe and unstable.

Topical cortisones in creams, ointments and lotions are extremely helpful for many patients with psoriasis. However, even these need to be carefully used to avoid side-effects. Side-effects include excessive thinning of the skin (particularly in the skin-folds and face area), and exces-sive appearance of blood vessels where the skin is thinned. At time this is very noticeable on the face. In addition, skin infections and hair follicle infections can produce problems with excessive topical cortisone use. Talk to your dermatologist about which cortisone you should use, and how. Generally, you will use the mildest cortisones, i.e. 1% hydrocortisone cream or ointment on the face, skin-folds and genital area. Stronger cortisones will generally be needed on other parts of the body.

Q: *I have psoriatic arthritis. Will my arthritis get worse with my psoriasis?*

A: Psoriatic arthritis generally does get worse following worsening psoriasis. There are a few patients who have psoriatic arthritis without any evidence of skin psoriasis. In general, however, they will develop skin psoriasis at some stage. Remember to protect the joints as much as possible when you have acute arthritis.

Q: *Will my psoriasis get worse if I am pregnant?*

A: Many psoriatic women who become pregnant do experience changes in their psoriasis. The psoriasis usually improves considerably during pregnancy. Unfortunately, it will frequently get worse in the months following delivery. If you are pregnant or likely to become pregnant, DO NOT use medications that can potentially harm the developing child. These medications include any of the internal medications such as methotrexate, retinoids and Cyclosporine. Additionally, it is probably unwise to receive PUVA

phototherapy or apply excessive amounts of topical medications. Fertile and pregnant women can usually use small amounts of topical corticosteroids, small quantities of Anthralin cream or ointment and as much moisturizer as they desire. Speak to your obstetrician about any medications you are using.

Q: *How common is psoriasis?*

A: Psoriasis is a very common disease affecting approximately 2% of the population. This means that one in 50 people has psoriasis or over 1 million people in the UK and 5–6 million people in the USA. It is often helpful for people with psoriasis to realize that there are many others with the disease in the community.

Q: *Should I wash with soap if I have psoriasis?*

A: It is best to use relatively mild soaps for any skin disease. Nondetergent soap substitutes may be less drying and less irritating. Examples of these soap substitutes are Cetaphil or Aquanil. In addition, soaps or bath oils that contain coal tars or moisturizers such as Balnetar or Polytar are very helpful as agents to soothe skin within psoriasis.

Q: *I am a 28-year-old married woman wanting to become pregnant. How can I treat my psoriasis in the scalp and body?*

A: It is wise to avoid any oral medicines, I can also recommend avoidance of coal tars and topical retinoids. I suggest . higher strength cortisone creams alternating with anthralin. Dovonex can be used. Moisturisers, ultraviolet treatment or sunbathing may help. Your psoriasis may improve during your pregnancy. (It may, however, get worse afterwards.)

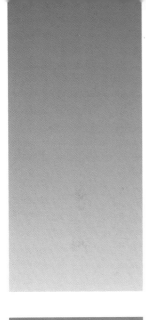

Appendix

Useful addresses of psoriasis associations for the psoriasis patient world-wide

Australia
The Skin and Psoriasis Foundation,
PO Box 228,
PO Collins Street,
3000 Melbourne

Belgium
Vlaamse Vereniging Psoriasis Patineten,
Heedstraat 33–1 730 Asse

GIPSO,
30 rue de l'Armistice,
4020 Liege

Canada
The Canadian Psoriasis Association,
The Women's College Hospital,
76 Greenville Street,
Toronto, Ontario

Canadian Psoriasis Foundation,
1565 Carling Avenue,
Suite 400,
Ottawa,
Ontario, K1Z 8RI

Psoriasis Society of Canada,
PO Box 9551,
Station A,
Halifax,
Nova Scotia B3K 5S4

Croatia
Dristvo Psorijaticara Hrvatske,
Svarcova ul. 20,
41 000 Zagreb

Czech Republic
The Society of Psoriasis,
Struharovska 2941,
14100 Prague

Denmark
Danmarks Psoriasis Forening,
Landskronagade 66.4,
2100 Kobenhavno

Egypt
Egyptian Psoriasis Society,
PO Box 29,
Citadel,
Cairo

Estonia
Eesti Psoriaasi Lut,
Kulmaallika 8A,
200026 Tallinn

Finland
The Finnish Psoriasis Association,
Fredrikinkatu 27 A 1,
00120 Helsinki

France
Association Pour La Lutte Contre Le Psoriasis,
1 Rue des Bois,
95520 Osny

Germany
Deutscher Psoriasis Bund EV,
Oberaltenallee 20A,
2000 Hamburg 76

PSO Aktuell,
Postfach 43 06 29,
D-8000 Munchen 43

Iceland
Samtok Psoriasis,
Og Exemsjuklinga (Spoex),
Bolholt 6,
105 Reykjavik

Israel
Israel Psoriasis Association,
PO Box 13275
Tel-Aviv

Italy
ASN,
Via Bergogne 43,
20114 Milano

ADIPSO,
Via Cavour 266,
00134 Roma

APSIAR,
Clinica Dermatologica dell,
Universita-341 00,
Trieste

Jordan
Jordanian Psoriasis Association,
PO Box 184 194,
Amman

Netherlands
Nederlandse Bond van Psoriasis,
Patientenverenigingen (NBPV),
Bouriciussur 4–6014 CW,
Arnhem

New Zealand
The Auckland Psoriasis Society,
PO Box 3062,
Auckland 1

Norway
Norsk Psoriasis Forbund,
Grenseveien 86 A,
0663 Oslo

Portugal
Associacao Dos Psoriaticos de Portugal,
1 Esq. Rhua Almeida,
Garrette 47,
8000 Faro

Singapore
Psoriasis Association of Singapore,
National Skin Centre,
c/o Phototherapy Unit,
No 1 Mandalay Road
1130

South Africa
The South African Psoriasis Association,
106 H Baker Street,
Groenkloof,
Pretoria 0181

Sweden
Svenska Psoriasisforbundet,
Sveavagen 31,
I1134 Stockholm

Switzerland
Schweizerische Psoriasis-Gesellschaft,
Postfach 8027,
Zurich

UK
The Psoriasis Association,
7 Milton Street,
Northampton NN2 7JG
Tel 01604 711129

Psoriatic Arthropathy Alliance
PO Box 111
St Albans
Herts AL2 3JQ

USA
The National Psoriasis Foundation,
6600 SW 92nd Ave,
Suite 300,
Portland, OR 97223

Venezuela
Venezuela National Psoriasis Foundation,
Centro Clinico Professional,
AV. Phanteon,
San Bernardino,
Piso 3, Consultoio 304,
Caracas.

Additional Sources of Information About Psoriasis

The National Psoriasis Foundation (NPF) is located at 6600 SW, 92nd Avenue, Suite 300, Portland, OR 97223, USA. As a member, you can receive numerous booklets dealing with psoriasis and related issues. For the cost of annual membership, which is a donation of any amount, members receive *Bulletin*, a newsletter that offers news on current treatments and research; educational literature —

numerous booklets on a wide range of specific topics; and *Pharmacy News*, a newsletter that announces new or unique products, lists over-the-counter and prescription psoriasis medications and also contains interesting articles. This publication is sent to members three times a year. These are just a sample of the items and services available from the NPF. The NPF can be reached by calling (503) 244 7404.

The Psoriasis Association in the UK is located at 7 Milton Street, Northampton, NN2 7JG, UK. Members receive their journal several times a year and may attend their annual conferences. It can be reached at 01604 711129.

The American Academy of Dermatology (AAD). The AAD has a consumer pamphlet on psoriasis that is available by sending a self-addressed, stamped, business-size envelope to: AAD, PO Box 4014, Schaumburg, IL 60168-4014, USA. Mark it 'Psoriasis'. The AAD also offers nearly 40 consumer pamphlets on a variety of skin and hair disorders.

The British Association of Dermatology (BAD) also makes available some patient pamphlets on different skin diseases. BAD, 19 Russell Square, London W1.

Index